RECOVERING
COMMON SENSE

RECOVERING COMMON SENSE

CONSCIENTIOUS HEALTH CARE
FOR THE 21ST CENTURY

C. Norman Shealy, M.D., Ph.D.

Sergey Sorin, M.D., DABFM

Amber Massey-Abernathy, Ph.D.

with poetry by
Georgianne Ginder

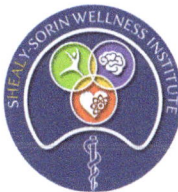

Shealy-Sorin Wellness Institute
Springfield, Missouri

Cover photo by A. Ogleznev (www.arthurogleznev.com)
Editing by JSB
Layout by Karen and Jesse
Library of Congress Control no. 2020923534
ISBN: 978-1-7362300-0-8

Common sense is the knack of seeing things as they are, and doing things as they ought to be done.

—**Josh Billings**

Society is always taken by surprise at any new example of common sense.

—**Ralph Waldo Emerson**

Science is a first-rate piece of furniture for a man's upper chamber, if he has common sense on the ground-floor. But if a man hasn't got plenty of good common sense, the more science he has, the worse for his patient.

—**Oliver Wendell Holmes, Sr.**

Common sense is in medicine the master workman.

—**Peter Latham**

[An] overall healthy lifestyle ... can be attained through common sense decisions about the way we eat, move, and live.

—**Harley Pasternak**

What is common sense isn't common practice.

—**Stephen Covey**

There is nothing more uncommon than common sense.

—**Frank Lloyd Wright**

Apothecary Shoppe

I've watched you rushing by—
Cell phone
Clutched in one hand
And in the other
Your coffee cup.

I see you too—
Those who live with pain--
Weary and worried
Feeling helpless,
Tired, almost ready to give up.

Healing is here
But we must stop
To see it;
Hope is here, too.
And thus we can be it.

For a minute—just a minute
Put down the cup and phone;
Depart from the flurry and from the fear
Because together in this healing place
We need not be alone.

—Georgianne Ginder (August 9, 2003)

Contents

Introduction

C. Norman Shealy, M.D., Ph.D.

This is not my first foray into conscientiousness in health care. In *Living Bliss: Major Discoveries Along the Holistic Path* (Carlsbad, CA: Hay House, 2014), I explored the implications of trait psychology for health. Back in 2014, I emphasized four "basic health habits" (p. 2): healthy weight, as measured by body mass index (BMI); healthy diet, including at least five servings of fruits and vegetables per day; adequate exercise, averaging 30-minute sessions five times per week; and no smoking. I've since learned to emphasize sleep—seven to eight hours daily— as a fifth habit. If you place these five health essentials at the core or axis-point of health, then "standing at the core" allows us to look outward at health's numerous encircling component parts. The philosophy of holism holds to the maxim, "the whole is greater than the sum of its parts." Here, the health essentials are like spokes connected to an axle encompassed by a circle. And that circle has become *something more*, something "greater than its parts." It's become a wheel: Call it the "wheel of life." In your mind's eye, see how its spokes, those health essentials, hold that wheel together. Whether it needs four spokes or five or six or more, the wheel *works*—holding us up, moving us forward—by the strength of its spokes.

And what of the axle, that axis-point that allows us to see health in its wholeness? Let's call it conscientiousness—common sense in action. Like a wheel, our health rides upon the five health essentials held together by common sense. Break one or two of these spokes or remove conscientiousness from the center, and the wheel falls apart. Conscientiousness, thus, becomes the axis-point of health care, holding us up and moving us forward by our commitment to the "basic health habits." If you understand this holistic metaphor, you will understand this book!

I take the term "conscientiousness" from Five-Factor Theory (FFT), as outlined by American psychologists Paul T. Costa and Robert R. McCrae. Within the Five-Factor model, the character trait of conscientiousness is joined by neuroticism, extraversion, agreeableness, and openness to experience: In varied combinations and degrees, these form the dominant traits descriptive of human personality. While FFT does not deny the uniqueness or individuality of individuals, the various traits are mirrored and replicated daily in one's actions, attitudes, emotions, choices, and responses. In this way, specific traits *typify* an individual, becoming predictive of behavior. Of the FTT traits, conscientiousness conduces to health, while neuroticism takes its stressful toll. The question arises: Are we "born into" our personality traits, or do we "grow into" them? If conscientiousness is the friend of health and neuroticism its enemy, can we choose one over another?

In their earliest iterations of theory, Costa and McCrae argued that "FFT does not admit of any influence of the environment on personality traits," for, "if traits are shaped by the environment, we should expect considerable change in traits over time, as most adult developmentalists did 20 years ago. But we find very little change. Therefore, traits *must not be shaped by the environment*" (*Personality in Adulthood* p. 152; emphasis added).[1] Additional research, however, suggested a more dynamic process:

> As it was originally formulated in 1996, FFT claimed that traits develop through childhood and reach mature form in adulthood; thereafter they are stable in cognitively intact individuals. By 1999, we acknowledged a need to modify that statement, because evidence suggested very small but consistent changes in Neuroticism, Extraversion, and Openness after age 30. (Costa and McCrae, p. 155)

Our own clinical research bears out this sequence: Personality traits, being genetically predisposed, "develop through childhood" and stabilize in adulthood. One's changing roles—as spouse and parent particularly—do impact the mature personality, as Costa and McCrae

---

1 On this basis, Costa and McCrae distinguished between "Basic Tendencies," which are "the abstract capacities and tendencies of the individual," and "Characteristic Adaptations," which are "concrete acquired structures that develop as the individual interacts with the environment" (*Personality in Adulthood* p. 151). Put simply, "Basic Tendencies" refer to the "big five" traits, to which individuals are genetically predisposed, whereas "Characteristic Adaptations" refer to the "interests, attitudes, beliefs, and the internalized, psychological aspects of roles and relationships" (p. 147)— which evolve over time and change with our changing roles. The former are innate, the latter learned.

suggest: "Perhaps at the start of independent life it is advantageous to be adventurous (open and extraverted) to meet potential mates and to learn one's way in the world. Once settled down, Conscientiousness might well be helpful in carrying out the routine tasks of daily life and Agreeableness might be an asset in bonding with children" (*Personality in Adulthood* p. 156). So, of course we agree with Costa and McCrae in looking for predictable, measurable growth in personality over one's lifetime. We disagree with them, however, in the limits placed on such growth.

We have two claims to make, both rather bold (though backed by clinical practice and experiment) and both making significant contributions to Five-Factor Theory. The first claim is medical: The FFT personality traits have hormonal expressions, such that openness, conscientiousness, extraversion, agreeableness, and neuroticism—the so-called "big five" of FFT—are mirrored in levels of dopamine, serotonin, acetylcholine, oxytocin, anandamide, and other neurotransmitters. We have not yet established the full neuroscience of FFT, but we have made a start. We know, for example, that individuals presenting high levels of neuroticism show depressed levels of serotonin and oxytocin. We also know that high scores in conscientiousness are reflected in high levels of these same neurotransmitters. It makes sense that gestation, birth, infancy, and early childhood contribute to the development and stabilization of personality, since these are the years of formative hormonal growth. In sum: FFT is grounded, not in genetics merely, but in our neurochemical pathways. Shifting metaphors, if genetics provides the blueprint, then neurochemistry provides the materials for construction.

Our second claim is medical as well, but turns from brain chemistry to patterns and habits of behavior. Personality traits—neuroticism and conscientiousness particularly—correlate with health and wellness. While FFT traits are genetic in origin and change slowly over time, it is our contention that one can, in fact, *choose health* by growing in conscientiousness. And, as we shall argue, the modalities of holistic medicine provide a means of growth. This book offers an outline of those modalities and of their role in conscientious health care.

In this sequel to *Living Bliss*, I've come to a larger understanding of conscientiousness. I used to see it as a personality trait operant in intrapersonal and familial settings primarily. Now more than ever, I've come to see its social, economic, and political implications. While *The Longevity Project* inspired my earlier discussion,[2] this present text takes inspiration from a text much older though no less revolutionary: Thomas Paine's *Common Sense* (1776). In *Living Bliss*, I argued that an individual's failures in health derived largely from the failure of conscientiousness; in the first chapter of this sequel, I look to the health of our nation and its

2 See Howard S. Friedman and Leslie L. Martin, *The Longevity Project: Surprising Discoveries for Health and Long Life from the Landmark Eight-Decade Study* (New York: Hudson Street/Penguin, 2011).

institutions of government, medicine, insurance, and academia. It's not the failure of any one American's health care that I'm interested in. It's the failure of *American* health care: the whole shebang. And, while the watchword previously was conscientiousness, the term for this text is "common sense"—or, rather, the lack thereof. For "common sense" has a rich history in politics and philosophy going back millennia but coming to a head in 18ᵗʰ century England, France, and the American colonies (soon to become the fledgling United States of America). I'd like to see some of that old common sense restored today.[3]

---

3 I take solace in Neil Postman's *Building A Bridge to the Eighteenth Century: How the Past Can Improve Our Future* (New York: Vintage Books, 1999). Postman writes:

> [I]n order to have an agreeable encounter with the twenty-first century, we will need to take into it some good ideas. In order to do that, we will have to look back to take stock of the good ideas available to us. I am suspicious of people who want us to be forward-looking. I literally do not know what they mean when they say, "We must look ahead to see where we are going." What is it that they wish us to look at?... If looking ahead means anything, it must mean finding in our past useful and humane ideas with which to fill our future.
>
> I do not mean—mind you—technological ideas, like going to the moon, airplanes, and antibiotics.... I am referring to ideas of which we can say they have advanced our understanding of ourselves[.] (pp. 13-14)

Standing two decades deep in the 21st century, I feel a heightened urgency in Postman's call "to turn our attention to the eighteenth century" (p. 17). For "It is there," he writes, "that we may find ideas that offer a humane direction to the future" (p. 17; emphasis in original), ideas "about inductive science, about religious and political freedom, about popular education, about rational commerce" (pp. 17-18). It is there, further, that "the idea of progress, and ... our modern idea of happiness" were invented, there that "reason began its triumph over superstition," and there that the universe was rendered "orderly, rational, and comprehensible" (Postman, p. 18). Such were the fruits of an age devoted to empirical observation, spirited public debate,

Let's think holistically, back to that wheel: What's true of an individual must be true of a nation. If American health care resembles a wheel, then *its* spokes are the hospitals and medical schools and pharmaceutical companies and insurance industry; they're the FDA and the CDC and the AMA. Oh, and did I mention government regulators and oversight? You think we're going to find common sense at the axis-point of *that* wheel? The onus of health cannot be placed on the individual solely, though the individual must, as a matter of course, take charge of his or her health habits and decisions. Put baldly, I've learned that the problems with American health care are systemic. And, just as Thomas Paine called for a political revolution back in 1776, so we're calling for a revolution in conscientious health care—a 21st century revolution that begins with the individual and that works in spite of, not by means of, mainstream medicine and its unholy alliances. That's enough preaching for now, but it gives a taste of what's to come.

I welcome Drs. Sergey Sorin and Amber Massey-Abernathy as my co-authors. "I" and "we" can be slippery words, so let me say that the "I" of Chapter 1 belongs to me. Drs. Sorin and Massey-Abernathy join me as the collective "we" of Chapter 2 (though, occasionally, we'll refer to ourselves in third person). Dr. Sorin and I join voices in Chapter 3. And Chapter 4, with its wisdom traditions ancient and "new age," I acknowledge mine. Throughout, I'm delighted to include poetry by Georgianne Ginder,

_____

and an exercise of common sense.

longtime member of the American Holistic Medical Association. Texts on health and wellness can get pretty stuffy, so Georgianne's poetry reminds us to feel as well as think.

There's a touch of folly in all this talk of "I" and "we." As a medical intuitive, I know that our thoughts and words are never entirely our own—nor should we want them to be. We are blessed by spirit-guidance. It is both humbling and exhilarating to know that the Universe watches over us and speaks through us. Though we sign our names to the byline of this book, our voices are part of that greater chorus of wise men and women who have gone before us and whose insights are woven into this text. A text is itself a verbal weaving—a textile of sorts—that brings various strands into a unity. East meets West. Science meets intuition. Politics meets personal responsibility. Body, mind, and spirit are brought into a conversation by means of this book.

Wisdom Walkers Old and New

Wisdom walkers old and new,
Then and now, timelessly true,
Welcome all—there is *joy* to do!

Ancient traditional wisdom,
If one can be so bold,
Need not seem ancient,... lost,... or old.

"Then" and "now" unite as one,
Harmonize in present time,
Co-create this Universe—
Sure, Secure, Sublime.

Despite such mayhem, deceit and rot
The wisdom path can be felt and taught.
Wisdom seekers, search and find
The holy path of the Divine—
The faithful tradition of humankind!

                    —Georgianne Ginder (August 10, 2019)

CHAPTER ONE

Common Sense: How Lost, and How Recovered

C. Norman Shealy

In its 1977 Winter volume, the journal *Daedalus* took as its special topic, "Doing Better and Feeling Worse: Health in the United States." Dr. John H. Knowles (1926-1979) introduced the volume and contributed its most memorable essay, "The Responsibility of the Individual."[1] Coming on the heels of our 1776-1976 bicentennial celebration, Knowles' essay (and the volume built around it) proved timely. His "Introduction" quotes the great Alexis de Tocqueville (1805-1859), whose *Democracy in America* (1835) made savvy observations on our then-youthful nation. "In America," writes de Toqueville, "the passion for

---

1 *Daedalus*, Vol. 106. No. 1 (Winter 1977), pp. 57-80. Before his untimely death from pancreatic cancer, Dr. Knowles was renowned as a physician, educator, and president of the Rockefeller Foundation.

physical wellbeing ... is general" (Knowles, "Introduction" p. 1). *I believe that.* Everything that I know and read about those revolutionary times tells me that wellbeing was a "general" pursuit, reflective of the new nation's commonsense pragmatism. In "the pursuit of happiness"— one of the core values inscribed in our Declaration of Independence—"physical wellbeing" might stand side-by-side with political freedom and economic opportunity. We were a practical people (as de Toqueville described us back then), and our pragmatism enabled us to thrive; and, to the extent that we *avoided academic medicine*—which, in the 18th century, regularly did more harm than good—we could look forward to a lifetime of relative health, given the land's fertile abundance and our ambitions to succeed. Besides, we had old Ben Franklin among other practical sages reminding us that "early to bed and early to rise makes a man healthy, wealthy, and wise." How commonsensical!

But Knowles, writing two centuries after the Declaration of Independence, sees an unsteady mixture of good and ill in the current state of health care:

> New knowledge is being generated about the hazards of drugs, faulty diets, and environmental contaminants, and the nation has shown its willingness to ban the production and use of certain toxic substances.

> And yet we feel dis-eased. We find intolerable the levels of deprivation and ill health suffered by significant

numbers of the American people.... While trying to balance public and private interests, maintaining the ideal of individual freedom even as we assert the imperatives of social responsibility and justice, we know that we are confronted with complexities that call for ways of thinking that are not bound to the old and exhausted ideologies of an earlier day. It is a new kind of pragmatism that is needed.... The challenge to the United States is to estimate correctly what reason, confronted by irrefutable facts, can accomplish, particularly at a time when something more than a reputation for humanity is called for. ("Introduction" p. 7)

His was a call-to-action, much in the spirit of our nation's Founding Fathers. The "new kind of pragmatism" that Knowles calls for rests in some sobering statistics. His essay, "The Responsibility of the Individual," reads as the State the Union's "physical wellbeing" in 1977. In 2020, we read the same stats and can ask ourselves, "Are we better or worse off, still?"

That "dis-eased" feeling that Knowles reported in 1977: Has it lessened? Has it stayed the same? Or are our prospects gloomier? "The health of human beings," writes Knowles, "is determined by their behavior, their food, and the nature of their environment" ("Responsibility" p. 57). Amen! Since our nation's founding, the history of health has been one of real progress in hygienic practice, scientific knowledge, and medical technology—progress that has accelerated over the past century, gaining speed with each decade. But, as Knowles observes, the steady advancement of medical science and the extended reach of "big government" in regulating services has *not* advanced our general wellbeing. For "prevention of disease," he writes, "means *forsaking the bad habits which many people enjoy*—overeating, too much drinking, taking pills, staying up at night, engaging in promiscuous sex, driving too fast, and smoking—or, put another way, it means *doing things which require special effort*—exercising regularly, going to the dentist, practicing contraception, ensuring harmonious family life, submitting to screening examinations" (p. 59; emphasis added). If Knowles is right—and I'm convinced he is—then any proposals to fix America's healthcare system must begin, not with science or technology, but with considerations of culture, politics, ethics, and psychology:

> The idea of individual responsibility flies in the face of American history, which has seen a people steadfastly sanctifying individual freedom while progressively narrowing it through the development of the beneficent state. On the one hand, Social Darwinism maintains its hold on the American mind despite the best intentions of the neo-liberals. Those who aren't supine before the Federal Leviathan proclaim the survival of the fittest. On the other, the idea of individual

responsibility has been submerged to individual rights—rights, or demands, to be guaranteed by government and delivered by public and private institutions. The cost of sloth, gluttony, alcoholic intemperance, reckless driving, sexual frenzy, and smoking is now a national, and not an individual, responsibility. This is justified as individual freedom—but one man's freedom in health is another man's shackle in taxes and insurance premiums. I believe the idea of a "right" to health should be replaced by the idea of an individual moral obligation to preserve one's own health—a public duty if you will. (Knowles, p. 59)

Knowles provides data on the relationships between health habits and longevity.[2] Though his criteria remain predictive of life expectancy in the 21ˢᵗ century, I have my own "big five essentials" for health. Note that each is expressive of personal responsibility in lifestyle or habit:

---

2 Knowles writes, "life expectancy and health are significantly related to the following basic health habits":

1) three meals a day at regular times and no snacking;
2) breakfast every day;
3) moderate exercise two or three times a week;
4) adequate sleep (7 or 8 hours a night);
5) no smoking;
6) moderate weight;
7) no alcohol or only in moderation. (p. 61)

Respecting longevity, his interpretation of these data is eye-opening: "A 45-year-old man who practices 0-3 of these habits has a remaining life expectancy of 21.6 years (to age 67), while one with 6-7 of these habits has a life expectancy of 33.1 years (to age 78). In other words, 11 years could be added to life expectancy by relatively simple changes in habits of living" (p. 62).

Normal body mass index of 18 to 24. Less than 30% of Americans have this "habit." Obesity is now the number one cause of premature death.

No smoking. Over 22% of people still engage in the number two cause of premature death.

Eat a minimum of five servings daily of fruits and veggies. The average American eats 2.2 servings. (And French fries and ketchup are *not* vegetables!)

Exercise thirty minutes five days a week. Only 10% of Americans do this.

Sleep seven or eight hours every night. Well over 40% of Americans fail this one. Those who sleep five hours or less have 1.7 times the risk of early death.

Here's the point: *Only 2.7% of Americans consistently practice all five essential habits.* And failure in any one of these habits increases one's risk of heart disease, stroke, diabetes, cancer. The average American dies twenty-two years too early through lack of conscientious health habits. *The most commonsense commitment in the Universe is to choose health!*

Writing some four decades after Knowles' essay, I've got more data to work with and a more sophisticated behavioral model to explain this near-catastrophic failure of health habits and lifestyle. Our DNA telomeres predict a human lifespan of one hundred possible years, whereas the American life expectancy stands at seventy-eight years.[3] To

3 See Troels Steenstrup et al., "Telomeres and the Natural Lifespan Limit in Humans," *Aging*, April 9, 2017, pp. 1130-1142. See also Ibø Østhus et al.,

be exact, it's 78.6 years for both sexes combined, according to a recent CDC report.[4] Whereas the life expectancy of women has remained steady at 81.1 years, the life expectancy of men has in fact fallen, from 76.3 years in 2015 to 76.1 years in 2016. You can blame the opioid addiction for consecutive years of decline, but that makes our point: A "bad habit"—and what could be worse than addiction?—robs us of life expectancy, *and* of liberty, *and* of our ability to pursue happiness.

Even when they know what's good for them, 98% of our fellow Americans "don't take their medicine." (Not all the time, at least.) Some patients, paradoxically, are wise *not* to follow the advice of their allopathic practitioners, since the medicinal and surgical "cures" often do their own damage. And it's not always an individual's fault. Some can't afford the medications prescribed, given the monopoly that the American pharmaceutical industry—the Pharmaco-Mafia, as I've called it—bleeds people's bank accounts, forcing them to choose between medicine and food.[5] That said,

---

"Association of Telomere Length With Myocardial Infarction: A Prospective Cohort From the Population Based HUNT 2 Study," *Progress in Cardiovascular Diseases* 59.6 (2017): 649-655.

4 See Kenneth D. Kochanek et al., "Mortality in the United States, 2016," *NCHS Data Brief* No. 293, December 2017 (https://www.cdc.gov/nchs/data/databriefs/db293.pdf).

5 Note that "pharmacy" and "pharmaceutical" derive from the Greek *pharmakon*. Though translatable rather blandly as "drug," *pharmakon* can mean both medicine and poison. It's a curious fact of pharmacology that many prescription medications work by poisoning some aspect of our complex human biome. "There's not one cancer that we cannot kill," I've heard an oncologist say, boasting of chemotherapy. "The problem," he continued, "is making sure that the patient doesn't die first"—from the medication. Readers should keep this ambivalence in mind whenever prescription medications are used allopathically: By its nature, the *pharmakon* is alternatively both medicine and poison.

many patients *do* receive wise counsel from practitioners, and a majority of *these* patients do not comply. They neglect their health, even when they know what's good for them. This is a failure of habit, of behavior—of personality—which needs to be called out and named for what it is: a failure of common sense.

And it's not just patients that are lacking in this common sense. Communities, industries, schools, government agencies and their officials are implicated in this failure. My co-authors and I have come to a conclusion, which we'll state up-front: Until we can restore common sense to the whole of American health care—to patients as well as practitioners, to the medical industry and government agencies tasked with regulation—we will never restore that "general" "physical well-being" that de Toqueville described as our nation's "passion" and birthright.

"There is nothing more uncommon than common sense." Frank Lloyd Wright once said this, but I learned it from my father and have repeated it countless times since. Still, I didn't know until very recently—June 26, 2019 to be exact—how deeply the failure of common sense was implicated in the failure of Americans' health. It was on that day that I started researching and writing this text, bringing in my co-authors as collaborators.

Ours is a crisis of individual responsibility writ large: Before resolving it, we must acknowledge it, name it, explore it, understand it. It turns out that we're dealing with a nexus of terms—responsibility, common sense, conscientiousness—that have social, political, ethical, and psychological implications. We'll unfold each of these terms one at a time, starting with common sense. That's one that our Founding Fathers would have used. It was present at the birth of our nation and bore fruit in our nation's youth, as de Toqueville implies. But, somehow, we seem to have lost it: Certainly we don't have much of it today. Still, an entire philosophy is invoked in this term, to which the next few paragraphs are devoted.

1. "We hold these truths to be self-evident ..."

Americans recognize and honor the words above. Presented to the Continental Congress on July 4, 1776, these very words declared our independence from England, turning thirteen disparate colonies into the United States of America. More than inspire us, words like these have much to teach us, still.

In our contemporary world of conflicting attitudes, motives, and interests, let's assume that consensus is still possible and that we can all still agree on something—on *anything*—each one of us together. Surely there are basic beliefs and principles to which we can all still give our hearty consent. "Life, liberty, and the pursuit of happiness," for example: Who among us would say no to these? Actually, our capacity for agreement shouldn't surprise; the authors of the Declaration of Independence took it for granted. They took it for granted, because their philosophy of government mirrored their understanding of the human mind and its workings. This insight needs some explaining.

The Founding Fathers thought and wrote and acted during that great age of Enlightenment, the 18th century. It was an age of Revolution as well, in the sciences and technology as in politics. And Enlightenment philosophy's favorite subject was human nature, which it subjected to analysis and critique—physically, socially, economically, ethically, spiritually, politically. At the time, two schools of philosophy dominated in the English-speaking world: the empiricist skepticism of David Hume (1711-1776) and the commonsense realism of Thomas Reid (1710-1796). In many respects, Reid developed his philosophy as an antidote to Hume's skepticism. Still, both schools—the empiricist and the realist—shared similar aims in seeking to understand *how the mind works*, and both developed a model of human consciousness grounded in "faculty psychology." Again, we need to explain.

Of these two Scottish philosophers,[6] Thomas Reid most concerns us, since it was his ideas that made their way across the Atlantic, inspiring the American Revolution. Reason, memory, and imagination are among our mental faculties. Our bodily senses—of sight, sound, smell, taste, and touch—form five more. And a further faculty unites these, mediating between mind and body and creating a unified consciousness. Reid called this unifying faculty

---

6 Both Thomas Reid and David Hume hailed from Edinburgh, though Reid's work—joined by compatriots Adam Ferguson, James Beattie, and Dugald Stewart—came to be called the Scottish School of Common Sense. Please note that ours is the merest pencil-sketch of 18th century philosophy. For a more detailed explication, see Sophia Rosenfeld's *Common Sense: A Political History* (Cambridge, MA: Harvard University Press, 2011).

our "*common* sense," common in that it brought all other faculties together into a synthesis of thought, sensation, deliberation, and will, and common in that *we are all born with it*. Further, this faculty is presumed to be *identical* in us all. Individuals might "use it" in varying degrees, but its proper functioning guarantees consensus, uniting its human possessors in a singular, knowable, sharable, communicable vision of the world. Such is the Enlightenment notion of "common sense." According to Reid, it's innate and it's the same in all of us, *assuming that we choose to use it.*

Of all our human faculties, common sense is the most practical: By its means, we are saved—literally on a daily basis—from countless accidents and errors of judgment. If you see a pot of water boiling on a stove, do you really need to be told not to stick your fingers in it? If you smell rotting fish, do you need to be told not to eat it? If you see a baseball hurtling at you and hear its sizzle through the air, do you need to be told to duck? Of course not. You'll need no urging beyond your own native awareness. "It's commonsensical," you'll say to yourself: "Only a fool would do otherwise." And what's a fool? Someone lacking in common sense ...

Ironically perhaps, modern philosophy pushes us away from commonsense realism into habits of skepticism. Sure, "common sense" is useful enough as a metaphor for sound judgment. But where's the empirical evidence that such an innate mental faculty exists? Consider the instinctual patterns in animal behavior. A new-born kitten will not step from a solid wooden table onto a plate glass when its eyes see a sudden drop-off: Its eyes say no, despite the tactile signals of its footpads. Note that this hesitation has nothing to do with the animal's prior experience: As a new-born, its hesitation is instinctive. Humans, too, have an innate capacity for self-protection: witness the "fight or flight" response that's hardwired into our nervous systems.[7]

We've made this brief detour through human-animal behavior, in order to put a more recognizably modern face upon 18th century faculty psychology. In a nutshell, Reid's common sense describes "an instinctual awareness" or, put in Jungian terms, *an immediate apprehension* of the world and self in its truths. *No one has to tell you* that you're alive, that the material world exists, and that you'd better duck before that baseball smacks you in the face.[8]

Whereas Hume's skeptic worried over basic categories of knowledge, Reid's commonsense realist accepted the foundational "principles" of knowledge as instinctive: that is, *as self-evident*. This last became a catch-phrase of 18th

---

7 Even our imaginations seem governed by instinctual patterning: The great Swiss psychologist Carl G. Jung (1875-1961) devoted his career to an analysis of "patterns of apprehension" within the human psyche, patterns which he termed archetypes of the Collective Unconscious.

8 In his *Inquiry in the Human Mind on the Principles of Common Sense* (1764), Reid writes, "If there are certain principles, as I think there are, which *the constitution of our nature* leads us to believe, and which *we are under a necessity to take for granted* in the common concerns of life, without being able to give a reason for them— these are what we call the principles of common sense; and what is manifestly contrary to them, is what we call absurd" (p. 33; emphasis added). To trust common sense is to trust our own biological nature. As Reid writes in *Essays on the Active Powers of Man* (1788), "the faculties which nature hath given us, are the only engines we can use to find out the truth," and "we are born under a necessity of trusting them" (p. 237).

century commonsense realism. Anything self-evident needed no justification and admitted of no debate, for its foundation rests in intuition—not in argument. Indeed, from a Jungian perspective, Reid's common sense faculty resides within the intuitive function *per se*, which takes "immediate apprehension" as its definition. (In later chapters, we'll have more to say on these terms, their definitions, and their applications to health.)

And now for the punchline: Our Declaration of Independence, arguably the most thrilling document in American history, rests in the philosophy of common sense: "We hold these truths to be *self-evident* ..."

"Life, liberty, and the pursuit of happiness" remain sacred values to all Americans in all times. Here and now, in the 21st century—some 244 years after these immortal words were penned—we continue this pursuit, though we seem to have squandered away much of our birthright. If you ask what enemies we face as a nation—what threats we face to life, liberty, happiness—the list is long. But we're not talking about foreign tyrants of the sort that Thomas Paine (1737-1809) excoriates in his revolutionary pamphlet, *Common Sense*. The tyrannies that we face are insinuated in our health systems and practices. We are an oppressed people, shackled to a broken healthcare system, betrayed by patent medicines and failed practices; and, perhaps worst of all, we have given up our own freedoms in the management of health care. Our forefathers and mothers overthrew foreign tyranny, and we've desecrated their memories by an oppression self-imposed. And addiction is our worst oppressor, though it comes in many forms.

As desperately as Americans in 1776, we need a revolution today, though it's in health that the crisis lies.

We declare that matters of health cannot be separated from those sacred values of life, liberty, and happiness, for indeed, illness robs us of these values. What happiness can lie in unrelenting chronic illness? What liberty is lost in addiction? What *quality* of life can we expect from our increasingly degraded environment? We wish it were as easy as saying, "Enough. Let's take health care into our own hands. Let's do in realms of health care what the old Revolutionaries did in politics." The problem is, *they* had achieved a sufficient political consensus borne of common sense. And, somehow, *we've lost that faculty.* We are no longer governed by common sense.

Though there's hope in regaining this faculty, it's not an easy fix. We wish it were as easy as writing a pamphlet—the holistic healthcare equivalent of Paine's *Common Sense*—and that readers would respond positively to our call-to-action. But, just over the past few decades, thousands of books and lectures and treatment programs and consultations have pointed the way to that greater health which remains foundational to our quality of life and ultimate happiness. Wise and well-intentioned, these efforts have failed to improve our collective health. The authors of this present text have concluded that the problem lies within. Believe it or not, *most of us already know* what to do to maintain health, live the good life, and achieve real happiness. We know what to do, but we don't do it. And we don't do it because we are no longer guided by our intuitions. In sum, we've lost our common sense. And, until we've restored this habit, both individually and collectively, we'll remain enslaved to illness and its ravages.

2. Fighting for Common Sense (and Sometimes Winning)

Here's a scenario. Say there's something insidious in the environment—in public tap water, no less—that has been implicated in multiple, serious medical conditions. A sampling of symptoms:

1. Hypothyroidism.
2. Autoimmune diseases.
3. Higher cholesterol.
4. Infertility in men and women.
5. Increased bursitis.
6. Osteoporosis.
7. Arthritis.
8. Decreased IQ.
9. Increased instances of Down Syndrome.
10. Increased instances of hip fracture.
11. Increased hypertension.
12. Increased instances of Alzheimer's.
13. Calcification of the pineal gland.
14. Decreased testosterone.
15. Increased instances of heart failure.
16. Increased instances of kidney failure.
17. Increased instances of liver failure.

18. Increased instances of cancer.

19. Increased learning disability.

20. Increased diabetes.

21. Lead poisoning.

22. Increased inflammation.

23. Increased indigestion, abdominal pain, nausea, and vomiting.

24. Seriously weakened immune system.

This "something" can be shown to impact the death rate nationally. *I assume that you want to know what it is*, since you'll want to avoid it like the plague and work to remove it from the environment. You might be thinking that it's lead from old pipes or some chemical waste that's been leaching for years into groundwater. In fact, it's fluoride, which the American Dental Association (ADA) continues to promote as an additive in public water supplies.

Think about that: Since the 1950s, the fluoride that local governments have added to tap water to reduce tooth decay turns out to be a slow, steady killer.[9] "Fluoridated water amounts to public murder on a grand scale," declared Dr. Dean Burk (1904-1988), award-winning biochemist and one-time head of the National Cancer Institute. Testifying before Congress in 1976, Dr. Burk stated, "In point of fact, fluoride causes more cancer death, and causes it faster than any other chemical."[10]

9 See Sheldon Krimsky, "Is Fluoride Really All That Safe?" *Chemical & Engineering News* 82 (2004): 35–36. See also Bette Hileman, "Fluoride Risks Are Still A Challenge," *Chemical & Engineering News* 84 (2006): 34-37.

10 Quoted in "Fluoride—Killing Me Softly," web accessed 20 November 2019 (http://pecangroup.org/educate-yourself/fluoride-killing-me-softly/).

fluoridation is, at the least, a major contribution to mental and IQ problems.[11] And fluoridation has reduced male fertility from 150 million to 40 million.[12] In fact, if local governments continue this ADA-sponsored poisoning, within a mere generation most American men will be infertile—*no more babies!* Forget having grandkids and great grandkids.[13]

Now, if people actually *want* to ingest fluoride, they can get it in toothpastes and some mouthwashes: People should be allowed that freedom to choose. Unfortunately, the government makes the decision for us: Pour a glass of public tap water, and you'll be getting your daily dose of fluoride. And the problem's more widespread than you might think, given the number of drugs that contain fluoride. These include Advair, Atorvastatin, Baycol, Celebrex, Dexamethasone, Diflucan, Flonase, Haldol, Lipitor, Luvox, Fluconazole, Cipro, Levaquin, Penetrex, Tequin, Factive,

For an extensive discussion, see Barry Groves, *Fluoride: Drinking Ourselves to Death?* (Austin, TX: Greenleaf, 2002).

11 A. M. Barbeno et al., "Fluoride Exposure and Reported Learning Disability Diagnosis among Canadian Children: Implications for Community Water Fluoridation," *Canadian Journal of Public Health* 108 (2017): e229-e239.

12 Shun Zhang et al., "Excessive Aptosis and Defective Autophagy Contribute to Developmental Testicular Atrophy Induced by Fluoride," *Environmental Pollution* 212 (2016): 97-104. See also Andezhath K. Susheela, "Circulating Testosterone Levels in Skeletal Fluorosis Patients," *Clinical Toxicology* 34 (1996): 183-189.

13 While American researchers still occasionally sound the alarm, the most extensive scholarship comes from outside the U.S. See, for example, H. Cohen and D. Locker, "The Science and Ethics of Water Fluoridation," *Journal of the Canadian Dental Association* 67 (2001): 578-80. *In Fluoride: Drinking Ourselves to Death?* (Austin, TX: Greenleaf, 2002), Barry Groves presents a British viewpoint.

Raxar, Maxaquin, Avelox, Noroxin, Floxin, Zagam, Omniflox, Trovan, Flufastan, Paroxetine, Paxil, Prozac.

Protect yourself from poisonous fluoride.

The first suggestion is, I hope, obvious ...

Do not drink fluoridated water! Note that a majority of bottled water is fluoridated.

Liposomal curcumin has been proven to protect the brain from the toxic effect of fluoride. It's not certain that it protects the rest of the body, but at least your most important organ benefits from this natural anti-fluoride essential!

Why start with this story? Because it illustrates the inequality of power between individuals and various institutional and political authorities that claim to know "what's good" for us all; and most of us, too often, believe them and comply, unquestioningly. It's hard to take responsibility for one's life when the Third Party—that technological-economic-regulatory cabal of government agencies, mainstream medicine, and the pharmaceutical industry—does it for you.[14] I've cited water fluoridation as a failure of common sense. In this case, part of the failure lies

---

14 As Gary Null et al. writes, "the medical environment has become a labyrinth of interlocking corporate, hospital, and governmental boards of directors and advisors, infiltrated by the drug companies (*Death by Medicine* p. 162). Such is the Third Party, as I'm describing it.

with government agencies that continue to ignore fluoride's side effects; but the failure also lies with "the people," who either don't know or don't care. Let me give you three more examples of common sense gone crazy at the highest levels of society: tyranny in the form of hereditary monarchy, state-supported slavery, and nuclear power.

Remember that we fought the American Revolution to rid ourselves of tyranny. Since when has a king or queen been proved to be wise, benevolent, or worthy of rule "by birth" alone? (Is there some "royalty gene" that I'm unaware of, one that DNA scientists have yet to discover?) It was by reading Paine's Revolutionary War pamphlet, *Common Sense*, that I was put on the path that led to this book—put in search, that is, for common sense in health care. Note that Paine's pamphlet was (and, arguably, still is) revolutionary *in thought*: His commonsense preference of freedom over monarchy inspired us to become revolutionaries *indeed*. (I'll have more to say about Paine shortly.)

And remember that we fought the American Civil War over the "politics of slavery." Slavery of any sort ignores the sacred truth that all people are God's creation. And we are "created *equal*," as the Declaration of Independence professes, though it has taken many generations to confer this same equality upon all men and women: To this day, our sacred freedoms remain a social-political work-in-progress.

As for nuclear power, its fate is a bit different. Whereas tyranny and slavery were meant to die in war, the atom bomb came to life in wartime—born in an explosion over the Japanese city of Hiroshima on August 6, 1945, killing upwards of 140,000 civilians (60,00 instantaneously in the blast, the rest by radiation poisoning). The atom is capable of destroying the planet, as we have no way to control it (or remediate it) once its full force is unleashed, whether in an act of war or an act of terror or by "natural causes" (earthquakes and tsunamis come to mind) or by human error. Just to name the more serious, there's been the Fukushima Daiichi nuclear disaster (2011), Chernobyl (1986), Three Mile Island (1979), and the SL-1 accident at the National Reactor Testing Station in Idaho (1961). There have been dozens more accidents of varying degrees of severity, both civilian (in power plants) and military (in submarines especially).[15] In the U.S., some sixty nuclear power plants currently provide one fifth of the nation's electricity, though aging facilities and increased construction costs are likely to bring those numbers down. Still, if every nuclear reactor in America were shut down today, their deadly radiation would abide for more than a million years.

Here's my point: Sometimes we've joined together as a people and fought for our freedoms, and sometimes we've scattered and given up. Nowadays, it seems that we do less of the former and more of the latter. These threats to freedom—tyranny and enslavement in its various forms,

---

15 For seminal discussions of the dangers posed, see Harvey Wasserman et al., *Killing Our Own: The Disaster of America's Experience with Atomic Radiation* (New York: Dell, 1982), and Charles Perrow, *Normal Accidents: Living with High-Risk Technologies* (New York: Basic Books, 1984). For more recent arguments, see Chris Clearfield and Andras Tilcski, *Meltdown: Why Our Systems Fail and What We Can Do About It* (New York: Penguin, 2018).

plus environmental toxins like radiation and fluoridation—are with us still, today. They demand our vigilance. But our lack of such vigilance is corollary to a lack of common sense. And that's the broad subject of this book: how common sense is lost, and how restored. *If* it can be restored, then our nation's physical, social, emotional, spiritual health will improve in turn; *if not*, well then …

I've got some "war stories" of my own to tell. In 1958, chronic spinal pain was often treated by cordotomy—an aggressive, risky neurosurgical procedure that disabled nerve tracts in the spine. At the time, this procedure required laminectomy: the opening and removal of portions of vertebrae. Wanting no part of this medical barbarism, I researched and experimented for the next nine years, seeking a safer, saner, non-invasive alternative. Pain, after all, is a bioelectric nerve signal sent across neural pathways to the brain. Rather than cut into the spinal cord and sever its pain receptors, I developed an electronic device that sought to change the nerve signal, flooding neural pathways with external electronic impulses. When I presented my research and instrument at the annual meeting of neurosurgeons, many rejected it out of hand for having been conducted and demonstrated only in animals. *The Journal of Neurosurgery* turned down the article I had written for being "too controversial." Two years later, I presented results on my first six human patients: This time, every neurosurgeon in the room wanted to do the procedure of spinal cord stimulation. Today, the principle of transcutaneous electrical nerve stimulation (TENS) is a medical commonplace, with TENS units sold the world over. That's an opening salvo, but we're still far from a holistic healthcare revolution.

In 1978, I founded the American Holistic Medical Association. I was saddened but not surprised that a former neurosurgical colleague of mine wrote an article attacking the movement's leader for being "too charismatic" and "speaking too well." "Besides," he went on to write, "we are too busy taking care of illness to try to prevent it." Common sense is indeed the uncommon commodity! Of course, his words spoke directly to the opposition between allopathy and holism, the former based in a disease model of health care, the latter in wellness and prevention. Back then, I had hope that a revolution— in holistic health care—was rising. Four decades have passed, and I'm still waiting for that revolution. Each year, a new cohort of medical students prepares to join our ranks; and each year, the Third Party pulls them back into the allopathic mindset of mainstream medicine. In a recent study, first-year med students were polled at a large Midwestern medical school.[16] A vast majority (84%) "reported that knowledge about alternative medical therapies would be important to them as future physicians," while an impressive number (72%) "wanted to learn about alternative therapies while in medical

---

16 K. A. Griener, J. L. Murray, and K. J. Kallall, "Medical student interest in alternative medicine," *Journal of Complementary and Alternative Medicine* 6 (2000): 231-34.

school." Yet a mere handful (6%) "thought they would receive adequate exposure" in school. This fits my own observations. By the fourth year of med school, maybe one in ten students have kept an interest in holism; after residency training, the number drops close to zero. The common sense is drilled out of them. Then again, it's drilled out of their patients, as well.

As I've written elsewhere, conscientiousness is the single most important personality trait for health, longevity and lifetime income.[17] In 2011, *The Longevity Project* reported an eighty-year study on 1,500 students who were rigorously evaluated over their lifetime; using the Five-Factor Personality Inventory, conscientiousness was shown to be the number one determinant of health, longevity, and income. Even a modest score in the upper 50% of the conscientiousness scale was critical to these most essential life qualities. Commonsense conscientiousness does not have to be 100% to provide health!

Some stats follow; you can tell me if these impinge on the nation's health. Children in America born out of wedlock: 40%. Marriages ending in divorce: 50%. Patients not compliant with physician recommendations: 60%. Patients not taking prescriptions as recommended: 75%.

---

17 In *Living Bliss*, I report on the following experiment: "Individuals were given propranolol (a drug used to treat hypertension, anxiety, and panic) or a placebo, and the conscientious people were much more likely to survive whether they took the placebo or the drug. In other words, the conscientiousness of taking it was more important than ingesting the drug itself!" (p. 26).

The Longevity Project. In 1921, Dr. Lewis Terman, a Stanford University psychologist, began gathering self-reported data on fifteen hundred gifted children whose lives were followed through ensuing decades. In 2011, Drs. Howard S. Friedman and Leslie L. Martin summarized the data in book form. In an appreciative review of their work (http://www.howardsfriedman.com/longevityproject/), Sonja Lyubomirsky writes,

> In 1921, before most of us were born, a remarkable study began tracking the loves and lives of 1500 Americans from childhood to death. The study continues even today, Incredibly, no one until now has chronicled and interpreted the findings from this monumental almost century-long project for the general public.

> "Is longevity associated with being married, daily jogs, living with pets, or faith in God?" Such are the sorts questions to which Friedman and Martin provide some rather surprising answers.

I've just mentioned divorce and conception outside of wedlock. Both contribute to a lack of nurturing, made worse when parents are mentally ill, alcoholic or drug addicted, abusive, or poorly educated. I calculate that only 2.3% of Americans are conscientious enough to take care of themselves, let alone care for their children! And a nation is only as healthy as its children. Don't forget, they're the ones who grow up, bringing their medical conditions with them. (The wheels turn: A healthy parent has a healthy child, who becomes a healthy parent in turn. An unhealthy parent, on the other hand ...)

These sound like moral failures; in some respects, they are. But a holistic approach sees more than morality. Let's look at neurotransmitters and brainwaves. How much of our nation's crisis in parenting reflects depressed levels of the "parenting hormone," oxytocin? People suffering from anxiety and depression show an increased asymmetry in the frontal EEG and little or no Gamma brainwave activity—nature's own best antidepressant. Love and compassion are associated with increased Gamma wave activity and increased production of endorphins, vasopressin and anandamide. Dopamine, serotonin, endorphins, and oxytocin are the body's "feel good" hormones. And when they're lacking or imbalanced: What then? Dopamine deficiency is associated with apathy and fatigue, mood swings, depression, decreased concentration, weight gain, and addiction. Other hormones have their effects, as well.

What if our nation's crises in addiction, anxiety, and

depression could be cured, not by drugs, but by brainwaves? The TENS unit, you'll remember, revolutionized pain management. At the Shealy-Sorin Wellness Institute, we've been field-testing the latest modalities in energy medicine. There's the Low Energy Neurofeedback System (LENS), Pulsed Electromagnetic Field Therapy (PEMF), and Scalar Wave—brainchild of the late great Nikola Tesla (1856-1943)—among other programs, systems, and devices. It's too soon to discuss these modalities in depth. By their assistance, hormones can be regulated and brain functions brought into balance. It might seem a bold claim, but we believe that people can lead healthier, happier lives by these means; increasing a person's conscientiousness can make for a more nurturing parent, a more caring spouse, a more efficient, dedicated employee. We have the knowledge and the wherewithal. What our culture lacks is the common sense to put it all in place.

Maybe we're lacking in something more than common sense. Maybe what we're lacking is the will to change—or simply to admit that change is needful. A person down-and-out won't get up until he's hit rock bottom: That's one of the tenets of Alcoholics Anonymous. Maybe that's what we need. To make for real change, we need to show where we've arrived as a nation: In our health habits, we've hit rock bottom. If we have the will (and that's a *big* if), we can fix the healthcare system in America. But, first, we need awareness.

You Are What You Eat?

If you're reading this book, I assume you know to stay away from "junk food," though you might indulge occasionally. If you're particularly health conscious, you'll try to avoid it all together. *But can you?* American agribusiness (the Food Mafia, as I call it) has reduced the health value and nutritional value of most of our food to mere junk: Perhaps 80% of the food sold in grocery store aisles isn't worth eating. So, it's not just our water, but our food that's being poisoned—and with the government's blessing. Through chemical fertilizers (typically too high in ammonium nitrate and far too low in magnesium), monoculture farming, and other technologies—which include genetically-modified plants or GMOs—American agribusiness produces more food per acre than the family farms of our grandparents; but, given the depletion of soil nutrients and pesticide poisoning, who would claim that today's produce is better than that of our grandparents? Don't be fooled by today's "big agriculture," which *seems* to succeed in supplying grocery stores with good-looking, firm-textured fresh fruits and vegetables year-round. This produce may look good, but it's deficient—and woefully so—in essential nutrients. We've known this at least since 1976, when Canadian biochemist Ross Hume Hall (1926-2003) published *Food for Nought*, which exposed the practices of modern agribusiness.[18]

_____

18 Ross Hume Hall, *Food for Nought: The Decline in Nutrition* (New York: 1976).

You might notice that the tomatoes sold in supermarkets stay consistently firm; that is, they don't spoil or "go rotten." By the same token, they're never really sweet—never like those garden-grown varieties many of us grew up with. Have you wondered why? It's because they've been altered genetically to enable mass-transport from hundreds and even thousands of miles away. Rather than ripen too soon, they're modified so that *they never ripen at all*. (Remember that ripening—which softens the flesh and releases sugars—ends in rotting: Ripening and rotting are one and the same natural process.) Again, the produce *looks* good when it arrives in the supermarket, but its nutritional value, not to mention its taste, has been sacrificed. (Actually, *we're* the ones being sacrificed, since we're eating GMO junk.)

And while "going organic" offers better nutrition and less contamination, we need to be honest with ourselves: There is, in fact, no truly organic food today, since much of the rain that falls on our nation's fields contains traces of Roundup poison (not to mention traces of fluoride). Since 1944, Monsanto (MonSatan, as I call it) has made billions off of pesticides like DDT and herbicides like glyphosate (i.e., Roundup): Having poisoned the nation's soil, Monsanto has genetically-modified numerous staple crops to make them resistant ... to their own herbicide poisons! These so-called "Roundup ready" GMOs have infiltrated seed stocks globally, making their human consumption virtually unavoidable. (Soy, some yellow squash, sugar beets, cottonseed oil and canola oil are at "high risk" for GMO seed contamination, but if there's one food to avoid nowadays, it's corn. The odds are nine-to-one that any American-grown corn will be "high risk" for GMO seed contamination.) We are still learning the health effects of genetically-modified crops that were introduced into our food supply—with government approval—in the early 1990s, but we can start with the following: increased infertility, accelerated aging, difficulties with insulin regulation, gastrointestinal stress, and a weakened immune system.[19]

---

19 "Genetically Modified Foods Pose Huge Health Risk." The Cornucopia Institute, 22 May 2009 (https://www.cornucopia.org/2009/05/genetically-modified-foods-pose-huge-health-risk), accessed 27 November 2019.

Note that these GMO health risks are in addition to the pesticide poisons for which these genetically-modified seed stocks were custom-made. The consumer website *EcoWatch* offers some unsettling news—the sort of news that the Third Party works to shield from most Americans:

> House-to-house surveys of 65,000 people in farming communities in Argentina where Roundup is used, known there as the fumigated towns, found cancer rates two to four times higher than the national average, with increases in breast, prostate and lung cancers. In a comparison of two villages, in the one where Roundup was sprayed, 31 percent of residents had a family member with cancer, while only 3 percent of residents in a ranching village without spraying had one. The high cancer rates among people exposed to Roundup likely stem from glyphosate's known capacity to induce DNA damage, which has been demonstrated in numerous lab tests.

See "15 Health Problems Linked to Monsanto's Roundup," *EcoWatch* 23 January 2015 (https://www.ecowatch.com/15-health-problems-linked-to-monsantos-roundup-1882002128.html), accessed 14 February 2020. Long-term Roundup risks include Alzheimer's disease, autism, birth defects, brain cancer, celiac disease, chronic kidney disease, colitis, hypothyroidism, Liver disease, ALS, MS, and Parkinson's ("15 Health Problems").

Flush poisonous glyphosate out of your body.

Note that the following is recommended for everyone as a lifetime habit. So, prove your level of conscientiousness and make this a daily practice:

Take one teaspoon of glycine powder twice daily for two weeks and then one-quarter teaspoon twice daily for life.

How did we allow this to happen? Our favorite poet puts it this way:

Insane Domain—
Haven't you heard?

Herd mentality:
Brainwashed banality.
Herd immunity:
Utility of community.

Forced vaccination:
Missed communication.

—**Georgianne Ginder**

3. Death by Medicine

One of the more recent assaults on common sense has been the so-called Affordable Care Act, but let's pause to consider how we got to Obamacare. Before the late 1920s, there was no medical insurance. Then two hospitals in Dallas, Texas offered schoolteachers twenty days in hospital each year for a Blue Cross annual policy of $6.00. That was the beginning of an insane policy requirement: Your insurance would pay *only* if you were in hospital. Ten years later, physicians serving logging and mining camps in Oregon began Blue Shield, again offering coverage for physician services in hospital. Interestingly, the initial reaction by the American Medical Association— the physician mafia—was to censure those physicians; but, soon, the physician-insurance-hospitalization combo caught on across the country. In the 1970s, a survey of physicians at Lutheran Hospital in La Crosse, Wisconsin, revealed that two-thirds of patients were hospitalized for no other reason than financial—so their illness would be covered by insurance. This century-old failure of common sense has paralyzed medical practice ever since.

In 1963, Lyndon B. Johnson pushed for Medicare. At the time, I was on faculty at the School of Medicine at Case Western Reserve University in Cleveland. I wrote a letter to the U.S. President, predicting that his proposals would bankrupt the country. The White House responded to my letter by siccing the FBI on me: For a week, the

Feds tried to have me fired from Case Western, their excuse being that I was a "communist." (Ha!) They failed, needless to say. In 1965, Medicare was implemented. Back then, medical expenditures constituted 4% of the GNP. By 1972, expenses had grown to 12%. Now, they make up as much as 20% of the GNP. Let this sink in: Today, one in every five U.S. dollars is spent on or invested in health care. And, today, skyrocketing medical bills are a leading cause of bankruptcy. Of course, the government has itself avoided bankruptcy, not by paying its bills but by increasing its debt ceiling—which, as I write, has topped twenty-three *trillion* dollars.

Government offices and Congressional committees often blame physicians for ever-increasing costs, but physician fees account for only 19% of total medical expenses. Rather, since 1965, costs have been driven by the Third Party: that is, by the collusion of government, the legal system, hospitals, the FDA, and the Pharmaco-Mafia. In the meantime, physicians have been effectively brainwashed into embracing the drug approach to health care.[20] It's what their clients want and have come to

---

20 Friedman's joke about "polypills" is no laughing matter:

> Back when the new scientific field of health psychology was just getting formally organized as a modern science, those of us interested in this new research used to tell a running joke. It was about polypills. It was clear to us that health was being "overmedicalized." That is, every human ill, vice, and failing was being turned into a disease to be treated by doctors, usually with pills. And, in turn, it seemed almost every problem was giving rise to its own government agency. (*Longevity Project*, p. 201)

expect: And why not, given the power (and ubiquity) of advertising? The pharmaceutical industry underwrites the initial research and drug testing; it patents and manufactures its products, sends its sales reps out to hawk its wares, and pours millions into publicity. "Talk to your doctor about X" is a refrain heard constantly on commercial television. And how are physicians supposed to respond? Will they tell their patients about the evidence *against* this-or-that drug's safety and efficacy? Will they even know the evidence, given the pharmaceutical industry's habit of suppressing negative publicity? As high as 75% of negative drug studies never see the light of day. (Remember: What gets published is what gets paid for.) And we should note that many "positive" drug studies have problems with reliability, though these go largely unacknowledged and uncriticized.[21]

Friedman continues:

> Just think, with enough pharmaceutical collaboration, we could swallow one huge capsule each evening and treat cholesterol, overeating, alcoholism, insomnia, headaches, aging, depression, shyness, sunburn, hypertension, inattention, inactivity, and erectile dysfunction, all at once!
>
> Distressingly enough, it now turns out that the joke was on us. (p. 203)

21   See John P. A. Ioannidis, "Why Most Published Research Findings Are False," *PLOS Medicine*, 30 August 2005 (https://doi.org/10.1371/journal.pmed.0020124). A nonprofit 501(c)(3) corporation, *PLOS* is a peer-reviewed open-access publication platform that accepts no advertising from pharmaceutical or device manufacturers.

Beyond problems with experimental design and sample size, the more insidious reasons for unreliability in research include cognitive bias (the desire to prove what you already believe), the "publish or perish" syndrome in academia, and the increasingly common practice of "paying for science":

In November 1999, the Institute of Medicine (IOM) completed its report, *To Err Is Human: Building A Safer Health System.*[22] The IOM's unsettling conclusion—that the leading causes of death in the U.S. are heart disease, cancer, *and the medical system* itself—spurred a brief if intense debate that spilled over onto the pages of *JAMA: Journal of the American Medical Association.*[23] In *Death by Medicine,*[24] Gary Null and co-authors Martin Feldman, Debora Rasio, and Carolyn Dean expanded the debate, arguing that incidents of death by iatrogenesis (that is, of illness or injury caused by medical treatment) are actually more than twice that in the IOM report—making medicine by far the number one cause of premature death. As Null et al. note, 80% of medical errors go unreported (p. 44). This is unsurprising, since physicians, hospitals, and the healthcare industry

---

when a lab is being underwritten by an industry or corporation, that lab has an implicit, vested interest in "serving its master."

22   Linda T. Kohn, Janet M. Corrigan, and Molla S. Donaldson, eds., *To Err Is Human: Building a Safer Health System. Committee on Quality of Health Care in America* (Washington, DC: National Academy Press, 2000), accessed 20 November 2019 (http://www.nap.edu/books/0309068371/html/).

23   See Clement J. McDonald, Michael Weiner, and Siu L. Hui, "Deaths due to medical errors are exaggerated in Institute of Medicine report," *JAMA: Journal of the American Medical Association,* 284 (2000): 93-95. See also Lucian L. Leape, "Institute of Medicine medical error figures are not exaggerated," *JAMA: Journal of the American Medical Association,* 284 (2000): 95-97.

24   See Gary Null, with Martin Feldman, Debora Rasio, and Carolyn Dean Edinburg, *Death by Medicine* (Edinburg, VA: Axios Press, 2010).

generally are loath to admit mistakes. (Acknowledged mistakes = likely lawsuits.) But consider that as many as 36% of hospitalized patients suffer medically-included injuries resulting in a 25% death rate. Consider, too, that 64% of in-hospital heart attacks are caused by patient reactions to drugs (Null et al., p. 47). These are just the tip of the Titanic iceberg of iatrogenic injury and death. Still, the actual iatrogenic death rate has been buried by various means, including death-certificate reporting. After all, it's the initial disease or injury that's listed as the *cause* of death in most cases, leaving the complications from medical intervention unnoted.

Does this mean you should not seek medical care? It is the opinion of the authors of this book that medical care should be sought in cases of acute significant symptomatic illness. In such cases, it can save your life. But, when dealing with chronic illness—that is, with an illness or a condition that has lasted six months or more (though you might consider your condition chronic if you're not better in three months)—there's often no known medical cure to begin with and you'll be facing a markedly increased risk of iatrogenic injury. In this regard, here are some all-too-common ailments and their typically failed treatments: Tell me if you see *anything* commonsensical in what follows.

Consider the research on prescription anti-depressants, much of which has been ignored or, worse, suppressed. (We've already mentioned several ways that research gets suppressed: Medical journals publish only what their editors approve, and those journals and journal editors are often beholden to the disciplines, industries, and special-interest groups that underwrite the costs of printing or purchase advertising.) Occasionally, the word gets out: Several recent articles, including one in the *New England Journal of Medicine*,[25] have surveyed the available research and lead us to conclude the following: If the many *negative* studies of antidepressant drugs had been disseminated, we'd see that the net cure rate for such medications approaches *zero*. In other words, antidepressants practically never "cure" depression; and while they may lessen the severity of symptoms, their side effects are powerful and virtually inevitable. And the suicide rate is increased among those prescribed such drugs.[26]

Hypertension—elevated blood pressure—is a chronic condition, indeed. Still, control of hypertension by the most common anti-hypertensive drugs is achieved in not more than 45% of patients, while nearly 100% of those treated experience some side effects; these include fatigue,

---

25 See Erick H. Turner, Annette M. Matthews, Eftihia Linardatos, Robert A. Tell, and Robert Rosenthal, "Selective Publication of Antidepressant Trials and Its Influence on Apparent Efficacy," *New England Journal of Medicine* 358 (2008): 252-260 (https://www.nejm.org/doi/10.1056/NEJMsa065779?url_ver=Z39.88-2003&rfr_id=ori%3Arid%3Acrossref.org&rfr_dat=cr_pub%3Dwww.ncbi.nlm.nih.gov).

26 As Peter C Gøtzsche writes, "It can no longer be doubted that antidepressants are dangerous and can cause suicide and homicide at any age." See his "Antidepressants and murder: Case not closed," *British Medical Journal* 358 (2017): 3697.

mental fogginess and, in men, erectile dysfunction. The effectiveness (and side effects) of hypertension drugs leads us to an even greater medical controversy: that is, to coronary heart disease and its presumed primary "cause."

For the past three quarters of a century, cholesterol has been named the enemy, and blood cholesterol levels above 200 with HDL levels below 50 are certainly correlated. There is, however, another culprit that is almost totally ignored: excess calcium. In 1991, Dr. Stephen Seely published "Is Calcium Excess in Western Diet a Major Cause of Arterial Disease?"[27] Appearing in the *International Journal of Cardiology*, Dr. Seely's paper ought to have raised eyebrows; instead, it's been buried, despite its rock-solid research. The ethnographic evidence is compelling: Coronary artery disease and hypertension are minimal in countries where daily calcium intake is between 200 and 400 mg daily. In contrast, the typical American intake is 1000 mg or more daily. It's *not* by statins or other prescription medications but by diet, exercise, and appropriate mineral supplements (like magnesium) that such conditions are most effectively managed. By the way, the popularity of statin drugs shows us the Third Party in action: Having "sold" the FDA on the safety of its products and having "sold" the mainstream medical community on their efficacy, the pharmaceutical industry begins

---

27   Stephen Seely, "Is Calcium Excess in Western Diet a Major Cause of Arterial Disease?" *International Journal of Cardiology* 33 (1991): 191-98 (https://www.internationaljournalofcardiology.com/article/0167-5273(91)90346-Q/pdf).

its massive ad campaign, selling statins to a nation now convinced of its need to lower cholesterol. After all, hypercholesterolemia is a disease, right?

In their web article, "Dangers of Statin Drugs: What You Haven't Been Told About Popular Cholesterol-Lowering Medicines,"[28] Sally Fallon and Mary G. Enig explode this myth:

> Hypercholesterolemia is the health issue of the 21st century. It is actually an invented disease, a "problem" that emerged when health professionals learned how to measure cholesterol levels in the blood. High cholesterol exhibits no outward signs–unlike other conditions of the blood, such as diabetes or anemia, diseases that manifest telltale symptoms like thirst or weakness–hypercholesterolemia requires the services of a physician to detect its presence. Many people who feel perfectly healthy suffer from high cholesterol–in fact, feeling good is actually a symptom of high cholesterol!
>
> Doctors who treat this new disease must first

---

28   Sally Fallon and Mary G. Enig, "Dangers of Statin Drugs: What You Haven't Been Told About Popular Cholesterol-Lowering Medicines," The Weston A. Price Foundation, 14 June 2004 (https://www.westonaprice.org/health-topics/ modern-diseases/dangers-of-statin-drugs-what-you-havent-been-told-about-popular-cholesterol-lowering-medicines/), accessed 28 November 2019.

Like so many other *exposés*, Fallon and Enig's essay is web-based. While the internet is often described as a "wild West" of unvetted websites and unverified claims, it's proven to be technology's great gift to democracy, taking medical information out of the hands of "experts" and giving it "to the people." Of course, one must always question the reliability and accuracy of sources; still, the internet provides both physicians and clients with access to massive data sets *that have saved people's lives*. Indeed, the internet gives individuals the ability to do their own research, checking on medications and their side effects and exploring alternative therapies. So I say, God bless the web!

convince their patients that they are sick and need to take one or more expensive drugs for the rest of their lives, drugs that require regular checkups and blood tests. But such doctors do not work in a vacuum: their efforts to convert healthy people into patients are bolstered by the full weight of the U.S. government, the media and the medical establishment, agencies that have worked in concert to disseminate the cholesterol dogma and convince the population that high cholesterol is the forerunner of heart disease and possibly other diseases as well.

The Pharmaco-Mafia's "success" with statins lies not in the drug's actual lowering of cholesterol, but in its popularity among physicians, who prescribe them like candy. To increase sales, the Third Party has consistently lowered its diagnostic measure, as Fowler and Enig note:

> Who suffers from hypercholesterolemia? Peruse the medical literature of 25 or 30 years ago and you'll get the following answer: any middle-aged man whose cholesterol is over 240 with other risk factors, such as smoking or overweight. After the Cholesterol Consensus Conference in 1984, the parameters changed; anyone (male or female) with cholesterol over 200 could receive the dreaded diagnosis and a prescription for pills. Recently that number has been moved down to 180. If you have suffered from a heart attack, you get to take

Instead of Statin drugs... If you're willing to risk muscle wasting or rhabdomyolysis, fatigue, restless leg syndrome, and a decline in cognitive function (among other side effects), then go ahead and take Lipitor as your allopathic physician prescribes. But if you do take a statin drug, you'd better supplement it with $CO\text{-}Q_{10}$ since statins deplete this nutrient, so necessary to proper muscle functioning. (Only recently have television commercials for statins begun making this vital connection.) And note that the longer you're on statins, the more likely one or more of their side effects will catch up to you. Here's our own set of recommendations:

Instead of a statin drug, you should take magnesium in adequate daily dosage, since this can counteract an elevated calcium level.

You should also take vitamin D3 in adequate dosage, since the average American is deficient in both D3 and magnesium. Inexplicably, many physicians recommend calcium with magnesium together. (Indeed, they're often combined as a cal-mag supplement.) This recommendation ignores the evidence that both calcium and fat in the intestines interfere with magnesium absorption. (For this reason, magnesium is more successfully absorbed through the skin than the gut.)

cholesterol-lowering medicines even if your cholesterol is already very low–after all, you have committed the sin of having a heart attack so your cholesterol must therefore be too high. The penance is a lifetime of cholesterol-lowering medications along with a boring low-fat diet. But why wait until you have a heart attack? Since we all labor under the stigma of original sin, we are all candidates for treatment. Current dogma stipulates cholesterol testing and treatment for young adults and even children.

Such is the allopath's love affair with pharmaceuticals. How about with surgical procedures and chemotherapy? When individuals elect to have coronary bypass surgery, some 95% survive ten or more years. That sounds like a success. Indeed, it's touted as one of the more successful major medical breakthroughs. But you pay your money and take your chances: 46% of coronary bypass surgeries result in long-term memory loss. Besides, individuals of similar age who elect *not* to have bypass surgery have a similar ten-year survival rate. (More than once I've thought to have "DO NOT OPEN!" tattooed across my chest.) There are some surgical procedures worth considering, but for men with an enlarged prostate, avoid any urologist who does not do Green Laser therapy. (Put simply, the TURP "roto rooter" procedure is barbaric.) As with most statistics, the survival rate following cancer chemotherapy is quite variable, but the five-year survival rate for cytotoxic chemotherapy adult cancer is 2.1%. Do you need more facts and stats of this sort?[29]

Here's the bottom line: U.S. medical expenses are the highest in the world. And yet the World Health Organization ranks the U.S. 37th overall in quality of health care—just behind Costa Rica (36th) and ahead of Slovenia (38th), Cuba (39th) and Brunei (40th).[30] The Third Party isn't doing well at all. So, what are we going to do about it?

4. The Holistic Solution

There is no true health care or even good disease care except in a truly holistic practice. The term "holism" was coined in 1926 by the South African statesman and philosopher, Jan Smuts (1870-1920), whose magnificent book, *Holism and Evolution* (New York: Macmillan, 1926), sought to integrate the disciplines of science, biology (and biological evolution), human consciousness, creativity, and culture. In popular parlance, we'd say that "the whole is greater than the sum of its parts."[31]

29 That's in the U.S. In Australia, the survival rate is just slightly better: 2.3%. See Graeme Morgan, Robin Ward, and Michael Barton, "The Contribution of Cytotoxic Chemotherapy to 5-Year Survival in Adult Malignancies," *Clinical Oncology* 16 (2004): 549-560 (http://www.ncbi.nlm.nih.gov/pubmed/15630849).

30 "World Health Organization's Ranking of the World's Health Systems," *Canadian Health Care Information,* 18 November 2019 (http://thepatientfactor.com/canadian-health-care-information/world-health-organizations-ranking-of-the-worlds-health-systems/).

31 Remember our wheel metaphor? It's all just wood and metal until you put them together. In his 2nd edition (1927), Smuts puts it thus:

The National Center for Complementary and Integrative Health (NCCIH), a U.S. government agency under the aegis of the National Institutes of Health, takes the following as its mission: "... to define, through rigorous scientific investigation, the usefulness and safety of complementary and integrative interventions and their roles in improving health and health care."[32] In *Energy Medicine: Practical Application and Scientific Proof* (Virginia Beach, VA: 4ᵗʰ Dimension, 2011), I list the ten major "Complementary and Alternative Medicine (CAM) approaches" as identified by the National Institutes of Health (NIH):

> The fundamental holistic [principle acts] as a unity of parts, which is so close and intense as to be more than the sum of its parts; which not only gives a particular conformation or structure to the parts, but so relates and determines them in their synthesis that their functions are altered; the synthesis affects and determines the parts, so that they function towards the whole; and the whole and the parts, therefore, reciprocally influence and determine each other, and appear more or less to merge their individual characters: the whole is in the parts and the parts are in the whole, and this synthesis of whole and parts is reflected in the holistic character of the functions of the parts as well as of the whole. (p. 88)

32 "The NIH Almanac: NCCIH Mission," 25 September 2019 (https://www.nih.gov/about-nih/what-we-do/nih-almanac/national-center-complementary-integrative-health-nccih). The webpage continues:

> The Center's top research priorities include nonpharmacologic management of pain; neurobiological effects and mechanisms as related to complementary health approaches; innovative approaches for establishing biological signatures of natural products; emotional well-being as a component of disease prevention and health promotion across the lifespan; innovatively designed clinical trials to assess complementary approaches and their integration into health care; and communications strategies and tools to enhance scientific literacy and understanding of clinical research.

1. Nutrition and lifestyle: diet, exercise, sleep, and stress management.

2. Mind/Body Medicine: including hypnosis and a wide variety of mind-focused approaches, such as meditation.

3. Alternative Systems of Medical Thought: Traditional Chinese Medicine (TCM), kampo, Tibetan medicine, and acupuncture.

4. Yoga, ayurvedic medical systems, Native American, and Yoruba-based medicine.

5. Alternative Systems of Medical Thought: homeopathy and flower essences.

6. Bioenergetic Medicine: evaluating the intrinsic body energy to measure and treat disorders.

7. Pharmacologic/Biologically Based: herbal medicine.

8. Pharmacologic/Biologically Based: nutrition, dietary supplements, and vitamins.

9. Manipulative Therapies: chiropractic, osteopathic.

10. Manipulative Therapies: massage. (p. 4)

Put these together and you have a comprehensive program for health.

In contrast, "divide and conquer" is the allopathic mantra. Mainstream medicine has fought vigorously against every competitor, including osteopathy, chiropractic, naturopathy, meridian therapy, homeopathy, and herbology. (In fact, most of the modalities listed above have been discounted, doubted, or undervalued at the very least.) And non-Western modalities—native traditions in particular—are rejected out of hand. As I write, there are millions more people being treated by Chinese traditions of acupuncture and herbology and Indian traditions of Ayurvedic medicine than are sitting in Western doctors' waiting rooms today. Billions, in fact, will live long and well without the Western allopath's services. And think of the horrors that knife-and-pill allopathy has left as its legacy: spinal cordotomy, frontal lobotomy, electric shock, and insulin therapy to name a few.

For a further example, let me return to a subject I've studied in depth: management of low back pain. Yes, such pain can be excruciating, even debilitating. Surgeries of various sorts, including spinal fusions, are the common "solution," despite their expense and general ineffectiveness. When, if ever, is such surgery warranted? Pain without weakness or numbness in the feet is rarely from a ruptured disc, and surgery for ruptured disc is virtually never indicated unless there is neurologic involvement. At least 25% of the time, such pain results from sacral shear or rotation, *whose presence is missed virtually 100% of the time* by MDs and even by many chiropractors.

If you as a reader experience chronic low back pain (or know someone who does), then this paragraph may be meant for you. Only a small percentage of DOs who do osteopathic manipulative treatment (OMT) or physicians trained by us in our Wellness Institute workshops recognize this disorder, which is completely correctable by a simple OMT procedure. Fusion of the spine is useful *only* when there is true instability or dislocation of the spine. And the use of metal and rods is an abomination: Simple bone fusion is far superior, being more "natural" and less aggressive, with fewer potential complications and side effects.

Another common cause of low back pain is arthritic degeneration of the facet joints (the facets allowing vertebrae maximum motion up-and-down and side- to-side). It's for this joint pain that many fusions of the spine are performed. In 1972, I introduced a simple and infinitely safer procedure, facet rhizotomy, which can be performed in thirty minutes or less. If someone is suggesting fusion of your spine, ask them if they think a facet rhizotomy would work. If they do not know what that is, run fast and find someone competent to try it. I personally have performed over 1,500 rhizotomies with no complications. A posture pump is a terrific adjunct that should also be considered before most surgical spine procedures. And various electrotherapeutic devices can help relieve pain, as well.

So much for back surgery. Hypertension can be managed 99.8% of the time without drugs, depression and anxiety can be managed almost 100% of the time without drugs, and chemotherapy for cancer is rarely worth considering. Atrial fibrillation is often correctible with magnesium supplements, and type 2 diabetes is well controlled almost 100% of the time with herbal and dietary approaches. With proper evaluation, chelation can prevent the need for coronary artery surgery. These safe alternatives to knife-and-pill allopathy are just common sense, that very uncommon commodity!

As the Buddha said, "Do not believe in anything simply because you have heard it; when you find that anything agrees with reason and is conducive to the good and benefit of one and all, then accept it and live up to it."

Returning to Thomas Paine: A Coda

> [A] long Habit of not thinking a Thing wrong, gives it a superficial appearance of being right, and raises at first a formidable outcry in defense of Custom.
>
> —**Thomas Paine**, *Common Sense*

Forgive this digression at the end of an already long chapter. It was my rereading Paine's pamphlet that inspired this book, and I wanted to give some deeper reasons why.[33] In describing the overreach of government, Paine's libertarian spirit remains relevant today. So I hope you'll take the time to grapple with his argument:[34]

> Some writers have so confounded society with government, as to leave little or no distinction between them; whereas they are not only different, but have different origins. Society is produced by our wants, and

---

33 In his Preface to the 3rd edition (1776), Paine writes, "Who the Author of this Production is, is wholly unnecessary to the Public, as the Object for Attention is the Doctrine itself, not the Man. Yet it may not be unnecessary to say, That he is unconnected with any party, and under no sort of Influence, public or private, but the influence of reason and principle." Beyond the author's continued pose of anonymity, he claims to be "under no sort of influence" other than "reason." By this claim, Paine aligns himself with the Enlightenment philosophy of his age.

34 I quote from *The Writings of Thomas Paine, Vol. 1. 1774-1779*, edited by Moncure Daniel Conway (New York: G. P. Putnam's Sons, 1894).

government by our wickedness; the former promotes our happiness *positively* by uniting our affections, the latter *negatively* by restraining our vices. The one encourages intercourse, the other creates distinctions. The first is a patron, the last a punisher.

Society in every state is a blessing, but Government, even in its best state, is but a necessary evil; in its worst state an intolerable one: for when we suffer, or are exposed to the same miseries *by a Government*, which we might expect in a country *without Government*, our calamity is heightened by reflecting that we furnish the means by which we suffer. Government, like dress, is the badge of lost innocence; the palaces of kings are built upon the ruins of the bowers of paradise. For were the impulses of conscience clear, uniform and irresistibly obeyed, man would need no other lawgiver; but that not being the case, he finds it necessary to surrender up a part of his property to furnish means for the protection of the rest; and this he is induced to do by the same prudence which in every other case advises him, out of two evils to choose the least. Wherefore, security being the true design and end of government, it unanswerably follows that whatever form thereof appears most likely to ensure it to us, with the least expense and greatest benefit, is preferable to all others. (p. 69; emphasis in original)

Paine's style belongs to the 18ᵗʰ century, so let's translate this text into modern terms. What he's writing about is the role of government *in shaping the behavior of citizens* for good or for ill. And there are two types of citizens, apparently. There are those who "obey" "the impulses of conscience" and are capable of self-governance; *these* look to government to protect their free exercise of conscience while seeking "protection" *from that second sort of citizen* whose subjection to vice threatens the prosperity and "security" of the commonwealth.

What Paine calls "conscience," we've learned to call conscientiousness. And the point that Paine makes for us—the reason why *we need to become revolutionaries in our time*—is that the qualities that make for health in the individual apply equally to the health of communities, professions, industries, and governments. We seek an American Revolution in health care, one that restores common sense to our life-choices and lifestyles, overthrowing the tyrannies of habit. But more than the individual needs reform: The institutions that are supposed to care for us have lost common sense, becoming tyrants in their turn. Undergirded by government policy, virtually every component of the American healthcare industry holds us in its grasp, squeezing us dry. And, insanely, the vast majority of Americans seem cheerfully to comply.

The common sense that we so desperately need begins with the individual: Such is the nature of freedom. But it must extend to the agencies of government as well, since their task, as Paine rightly notes, is to protect freedoms and provide security. I can do no better than advise readers to return to Paine's text as providing a roadmap for our own 21st century American Revolution in health care. In the meantime, let me sketch out his major premises; for these reflect the premises underlying our own present argument.

Following the 18th-century Enlightenment philosopher, Jean-Jacques Rousseau (1712-1778), Paine builds his political philosophy upon a definition of humankind: Ideally, a government should suit itself to our own human nature, enhancing our strengths while mitigating our weaknesses. *What would such a government look like?* Then as now, it doesn't exist; so we have to imagine it. That's what Rousseau did in his *Social Contract* (1762). Laying aside the reigning social-political structures of Bourbon France, Rousseau engaged readers in a thought-experiment, restoring humankind to its original "state of nature" and asking what sort of "cooperation agreements" (or *social contract*, in Rousseau's language) would promote freedom and security, both individually and collectively. The culminating insight of Rousseau's thought-experiment would inspire America's Founding Fathers in their rebellion against the English monarchy: In sum, the original social contract must have been freely entered into, such that government is *by consent of the governed.*

Now, Paine certainly read Rousseau. But he didn't feel the need to go back as far as to Adam and Eve. Instead,

Paine's thought-experiment reconstructs the circumstances facing New England's earliest European settlers. If they had worked individually to survive on their own, Paine's Puritan ancestors didn't stand a chance. But, by freely and conscientiously sharing labors, they had a shot at survival:

> In order to gain a clear and just idea of the design and end of government, let us suppose a small number of persons settled in some sequestered part of the earth, unconnected with the rest; they will then represent the first peopling of any country, or of the world. *In this state of natural liberty, society will be their first thought.* A thousand motives will excite them thereto; the strength of one man is so unequal to his wants, and his mind so unfitted for perpetual solitude, that he is soon obliged to seek assistance and relief of another, who in his turn requires the same. Four or five united would be able to raise a tolerable dwelling in the midst of a wilderness, but one man might labour out the common period of life without accomplishing anything; when he had felled his timber he could not remove it, nor erect it after it was removed; hunger in the meantime would urge him to quit his work, and every different want would call him a different way. Disease, nay even misfortune, would be death; for though neither might be mortal, yet either would disable him from living, and reduce him to a state in which he might rather be said to perish than to die.

Thus necessity, like a gravitating power, would soon form our newly arrived emigrants into society, the reciprocal blessings of which would supersede, and render the obligations of law and government unnecessary while they remained perfectly just to each other; but as nothing but Heaven is impregnable to vice, it will unavoidably happen that in proportion as they surmount the first difficulties of emigration, which bound them together in a common cause, they will begin to relax in their duty and attachment to each other: and this remissness will point out the necessity of establishing some form of government to supply the defect of moral virtue. (*Common Sense* p. 70; emphasis added)

Humankind, Paine tells us, is born in a "state of natural liberty," but the "wilderness" and its hardships—solitude, hunger, exhaustion—drive people "to seek assistance and relief of [one] another." If people acted in mutual assistance, "law and government" would be "unnecessary." People would, in effect, be a law unto themselves—they would be governed, in effect, *by common sense*. Yet a "defect" arises in human nature, one expressed in "remissness"— *in a failure of conscientiousness*, one might say. The sad necessity of government, thus, is to counter people's tendencies "to relax in their duty," both to themselves and to the community at large.

Paine continues, turning his imaginary commonwealth into an idealized version of the Continental Congress:

> If the colony continue increasing, it will become necessary to augment the number of representatives, and that the interest of every part of the colony may be attended to, it will be found best to divide the whole into convenient parts, each part sending its proper number: and that the elected might never form to themselves an interest separate from the electors, prudence will point out the propriety of having elections often: because as the elected might by that means return and mix again with the general body of the electors in a few months, their fidelity to the public will be secured by the prudent reflection of not making a rod for themselves. And as this frequent interchange will establish a common interest with every part of the community, they will mutually and naturally support each other, and on this, (not on the unmeaning name of king,) depends the strength of government, and the happiness of the governed.
>
> Here then is the origin and rise of government; namely, a mode rendered necessary by the inability of moral virtue to govern the world; here too is the design and end of government, viz. freedom and security. And however our eyes may be dazzled with show, or our ears deceived by sound; however prejudice may warp our wills, or interest darken our understanding, the

simple voice of nature and reason will say, 'tis right. (p. 71)

As if rehearsing the opening of the Declaration of Independence, Paine grounds right government in "freedom," "security," and "the happiness of the governed." These aims are affirmed by "the simple voice of nature and reason": that is, *by common sense.* In noting the "inability of moral virtue to govern the world," Paine is effectively declaring the failure of personal responsibility—which, here as elsewhere, we're translating as conscientiousness. (Where an internalized responsiveness fails, the external force of law compels.) Freedom, like common sense, is innate. But, just because you *have* common sense doesn't mean that you *use* common sense. That's why Paine wrote his pamphlet: to reawaken this slumbering faculty. For one thing is certain, in Paine's lifetime as well as our own: The failure of common sense costs us freedom.

There are two types of tyranny lurking in Paine's text, one belonging to the individual, one belonging to the state: The former is an internal tyranny of "remissness," bad habit, and vice generally, while the latter is an external tyranny, whether of foreign lords, an absolutist monarch, or a home-grown dictator, power-hungry and out for personal gain. Note that the former ("remissness") leads to the latter (tyranny). It's the same today. That's why Thomas Paine's *Common Sense* remains a vital text for the 21st century.

Small world and no coincidences

Madness in the labs—
Ethics and morality?
Virtual duality—
Science without God?
Akin to bait without a rod.

Swimming mindlessly are so many rudderless and ruthless soul-starved hungry souls.

A world of unchecked and disconnected dislocated lost sheep ...

A plague may be around the bend with all this mayhem.

—Georgianne Ginder

CHAPTER TWO

Conscientiousness, Personal Health, and Personality

C. Norman Shealy, Sergey Sorin, M.D.,
and Amber Massey-Abernathy, Ph.D.

Gnothi se auton were Greek words inscribed over the Oracle's temple at Delphi: "Know thyself." This ancient exhortation remains relevant today. More than our highest moral-spiritual goal, self-knowledge lies at the foundation of conscientious health care. It's the aim of this chapter to provide readers with tools for a deepening exploration, and understanding, of the self in its various components.

At the Shealy-Sorin Wellness Institute, we understand that health rests in the dynamic unity of body, mind, emotion, and spirit. We understand, further, that *diagnosis is a dialogue* between physician and client. There's lab testing and other detective work on the practitioner's part, but these can come later. First, *the client must tell his or her story.* Of course, clients can only speak what they feel or believe or remember. As they speak of their condition, they'll get some things right and other things wrong and leave out salient details: Such is human nature. Often, a client's understanding of his or her medical condition is focused narrowly on pain or fatigue or weight gain (or weight loss). To gain a fuller picture, *we begin by asking questions*—the more and more varied, the better. And, until we gain insight into their condition, we'll hope that clients' answers on questionnaires are honest and complete.

The Problem of Self-Reporting.

In a recent study conducted by Dr. Massey-Abernathy, personality was assessed through the FFT "big five" personality trait inventory (these being neuroticism, extraversion, agreeableness, conscientiousness, and openness to experience). Test subjects filled out questionnaires about themselves. They also had three other people—a family member, a close friend, and a stranger— fill out the inventory on their behalf. Results were eye-opening. Subjects reported themselves differently than family members reported them on all five traits. Compared to their friends' assessments, subjects reported themselves differently on four of the five (the exception being openness). Looking more deeply into the results, it appears that family members and friends reported the test subjects as "better off" than the subjects reported themselves.

Self-reports showed higher levels of neuroticism, lower extraversion, higher openness, lower agreeableness, and lower conscientiousness. Another interesting finding was that strangers agreed with the subjects' self-reporting more consistently than family members or friends, particularly on the traits of extraversion, agreeableness, and conscientiousness.

So, are we seeing ourselves clearly? Or do others see us more accurately than we see ourselves? The answer is a little bit of "both of the above." Within the FFT model, self-reports are most often used because personality is all about the person. *Who knows you better than you?* We tend to know if we're anxious, sociable, responsible, etc. There are times, however, when we speak and act differently—when we adjust "who we are" to where we are or who we're with. This is why social context is important in gauging one's personality type. You might be more agreeable to friends than to most strangers, or more conscientious to parents than to friends. So, it's important to look at all your roles or "social selves" and average your tendencies, so you get the best overall picture of your personality and its dominant traits.

Although self-report methods aid in identifying an individual's dreams and aspirations, they can be problematic when topics turn tense or embarrassing. There are aspects of self that are hard to admit, not just to others but to oneself. We might not answer questionnaires truthfully, particularly on matters of mental and physical health. We might want to appear better than we actually are, especially when someone else is viewing our results. We might be seeking approval through our results. We might be comparing our personality to others and, for that reason, not seeing ourselves as we truly are. And we are not always conscious of such misrepresentations. Any number of "psychological defenses" might keep us from admitting hard truths about the self. There's denial: "I can quite whenever I want" is the addict's typical refrain, obviously self-deceiving and self-defeating. There's repression, a convenient "forgetting" of harmful or shameful events and details. And there's projection, when we attribute negative aspects of our personality to those around us or to things outside our control. ("I didn't do that. *You* did it!")

For these reasons, it's good to get multiple reports on a person's personality. That means not only reporting for yourself but seeing how family, friends, and strangers rate you, as well.

1. Self-Assessing Health: "Let's get started ..."

Within the FFT model, conscientiousness is the single personality trait that determines *lifetime* health, happiness, wealth, and longevity. So, let's do a quick self-rating:

On a scale of 0 to 100, how organized are you?
Your response: _____

On a scale of 0 to 100, how responsible are you?
Your response: _____

We'll assume that you've given yourself a respectable rating on each: not 100 by any means, but somewhere around 75 if you're like most people who come to our Wellness Institute. Now, let's return to the five health essentials as outlined in the beginning of this book. *And be honest!*

> Do you have a body mass index (BMI) between 18 and 24?
> *If not—if you're above 24 in BMI—then deduct 10 points from both scores above.*
>
> Do you smoke?
> *If you do, deduct 10 points from both scores.*
>
> Do you eat at least five servings of fruits and veggies daily?
> *If not, deduct 10 points from both scores.*
>
> Do you exercise at least 30 minutes five or more days a week?
> *If not, deduct 10 points from both scores.*
>
> Do you sleep seven or eight hours each night?
> *If not, deduct 10 points from both scores.*

In *Living Bliss*, his first book-length exploration of conscientious health care, Dr. Shealy wrote the following:

> What is it that conscientious people care about, and why should *you* care? Well, these individuals

are pretty easy to recognize. They are prepared, neat, and orderly. They like things scheduled, and *they approach tasks in a focused, organized, and disciplined manner.* Conscientious individuals are careful, thorough, reliable, persistent, and prudent; it may sound a bit boring to some of you, but all these traits are good to have if you want to live a long and healthy life. Conscientious people are particularly resilient when life gives them big challenges that must be faced. *But the most critical aspect of conscientiousness is responsibility*; they do not blame others for their own problems. It is responsibility for self that is the cornerstone, and it leads a person to become stronger in all other aspects of conscientiousness. (p. 9; emphasis added)

As noted above, organization and responsibility are key components of conscientiousness. And conscientiousness, as we'll be repeating time and again, is predictive of health: The more you have of one, the more you'll likely have of the other. And health contributes to happiness, which contributes to longevity...

We've already mentioned Friedman and Martin's *Longevity Project*, which summarized the longest organized psychological study to date. Begun in 1921, its eighty-year evaluation of 1,500 ten- and eleven-year-old children reached some compelling conclusions relevant to FFT. It comes as no surprise that health, longevity, and lifetime income correlate strongly with conscientiousness. In contrast, low conscientiousness correlates with alcohol and drug abuse, tobacco use, obesity and lack of exercise, risky driving, risky sexual behavior, increased stress, difficulties in relationships, divorce, poor parenting skills, anger leading to violence (with increased rates of suicide), and early death.

As a precursor to FFT, German personality theorist Hans Eysenck (1916-1997) pointed to the ways that neuroticism and its trait aspects—anger, anxiety, depression—lead to illness and early death. Within a two-decade study covering some 3,563 cases, Eysenck gathered some gloomy stats: 75% of those who died of heart disease had lifelong anger, 15% had lifelong depression, and 9% had lifelong both! Of those whom we'd deem self-actualized on a Maslovian scale, only 0.8% died of heart disease.[1] Their positive personality must surely have given them "the will to live," as Austrian psychoanalyst, Arnold A. Hutschnecker (1898-2000), puts it in his wonderful book.[2]

1 H. L. Eysenck, B. Grossarth-Maticek, and J. G. Boyle, "Method of test administration as a factor in test validity: The use of a personality questionnaire in the prediction of cancer and coronary heart disease," *Behaviour Research and Therapy* 33 (1995): 705-10. See also his seminal work, *Smoking, Health, and Cancer* (London: Cox and Wyman, 1965). Though Eysenck's silent connections to the tobacco industry have recently come to light (casting a shadow over his claims), we do not doubt his insight. For further discussion, see Dr. Shealy's *Conversations with G: A Physician's Encounter with Heaven* (Bloomington, IN: Balboa Press, 2018).

2 See Arnold A. Hutschnecker, *The Will to Live* (New York: Prentice Hall, 1951).

The Five-Factor Model of Personality: The five basic traits or dispositions—neuroticism, agreeableness, extraversion, conscientiousness, and openness to experience—have negative and positive aspects sorted in pairs. People possess these traits in varying degrees, which various inventories and assessment instruments aim to measure. In Personality in Adulthood: A Five-Factor Theory Perspective, 2nd ed. (London: Guildford Press, 2003), Paul T. Costa and Robert R. McCrae give the following chart (p. 2):

Neuroticism
  Calm—Worrying
  Even-Tempered—Temperamental
  Self-Satisfied—Self-pitying
  Comfortable—Self-conscious
  Unemotional—Emotional
  Hardy—Vulnerable

Agreeableness
  Ruthless—Softhearted
  Suspicious—Trusting
  Stingy—Generous
  Antagonistic—Acquiescent
  Critical—Lenient
  Irritable—Good-natured

Extraversion
  Reserved—Affectionate
  Loner—Joiner
  Quiet—Talkative
  Sober—Fun-loving
  Unfeeling—Passionate

Conscientiousness
  Negligent—Conscientious
  Lazy—Hardworking
  Disorganized—Well-organized
  Late—Punctual
  Quitting—Persevering

Openness to Experience
  Down-to-earth—Imaginative
  Uncreative—Creative
  Conventional—Original
  Prefer routine—Prefer variety
  Uncurious—Curious
  Conservative—Liberal

2. Personality Trait Theory, Explained

The study of personality has evolved as an aspect of humanistic psychology (as opposed to experimental psychology and behaviorism). As we've seen, personality psychology places its primary emphasis upon traits: those distinctive qualities that mark or *typify* individuals. In the English language, there over 20,000 trait adjectives. Obviously, we can't use all 20,000 terms in characterizing an individual; additionally, not all trait adjectives are unique markers of personality. (Words work in clusters, after all: joyous, blissful, cheerful, merry, sunny, blithe, and many other words are synonymous for *happy*.) Therefore, researchers have worked from hypotheses, statistics, and language-based sample inventories/questionnaires in determining which traits are most important in personality. The Five-Factor model has been confirmed by dozens of researchers using different samples from different countries in different languages and in different formats. Its "big five" traits follow.

Neuroticism: This describes a personality that is maladaptive in its coping mechanisms and subject to increased stress. Individuals showing high levels of neuroticism experience more mood swings and emotional ups-and-downs; they also tend to have relationship problems. It doesn't surprise that neuroticism underlies many physical as well as emotional health problems.

Agreeableness: This describes a personality that is prosocial and empathetic. Individuals showing high levels of agreeableness are good at "reading" people's minds and feelings; they're skilled at negotiating to resolve conflict and are inclined to withdraw from conflict. Conversely, an increased empathy can weaken one's emotional and physical boundaries, leading to codependency and a sense of being overtaken—indeed, overwhelmed—by another's problems (which can lead to increased stress and even to a decrease in immune functioning).

Extraversion: This describes a personality that seeks frequent social interaction. Individuals showing high levels of extraversion bask in attention, excel at leadership, and show higher commitment to work; they also enjoy increased job satisfaction and overall happiness. On the negative side, an extraverted personality can incline to risk-taking (as, for example, a tendency to speed while driving leads to more accidents and road fatalities).

Openness: This describes a personality that is receptive to new ideas and experiences. Individuals showing high levels of openness have vivid dreams; they're adept at problem-solving and show less prejudice than other types. On the negative side, people of this type are more susceptible to extramarital affairs and have difficulty ignoring previous negative stimuli.

Conscientiousness: This describes a personality that is organized, responsible, and dutiful. Individuals showing high levels of conscientious are reliant, resilient, and industrious; being capable of "delaying gratification," they're good at goal-setting and task-completion. It should not surprise that conscientious individuals tend to enjoy better physical and emotional health, higher work attainment, and better relationships (particularly among dating couples). FFT gives a further outline of trait aspects reflected in conscientiousness. Five of these follow.

Self-Efficacy: Self-efficacy describes one's ability to set and accomplish goals. High scorers believe they have the intelligence, drive, and self-control necessary for achieving success. Low scorers do not feel as effective and may sense that they are not in control of their lives.

Orderliness: Individuals scoring high in orderliness are well-organized. They like to live according to routines and schedules, keeping lists and making plans. Low scorers tend to be disorganized and scattered in focus.

Dutifulness: Dutifulness reflects the strength of a person's sense of personal responsibility and obligation. High scorers have a strong sense of morals, believing it important to follow rules and keep promises. Low scorers find contracts, rules, and regulations overly confining and are likely to be seen as unreliable or even irresponsible.

Achievement-Striving: Achievement-striving individuals are goal-driven and strive for excellence. They have a strong sense of direction in life and choose lofty goals (though extremely high scorers may become single-minded, even obsessed with their work). Low scorers are content to get by with minimal effort and may be seen by others as lazy.

Self-Discipline: This trait aspect—also called will power—reflects the strength of one's persistence at difficult/ unpleasant tasks until these are completed. People who score high in self-discipline are able to overcome their reluctance to begin tasks and will stay "on track" despite distractions.

Although all these traits have some impact on our emotional and physical health, research has shown that conscientiousness plays one of the biggest roles in *all* areas of life. Individuals scoring high in conscientiousness engage in fewer risky health behaviors; they have lower BMIs and show fewer behavior problems (such as deviance, suicide attempts, substance abuse, prison stays, and antisocial acts). Conscientious people are also better at sticking to exercise plans, choosing healthful foods and monitoring food intake, following nutrition guidelines, and reducing stress. Success and satisfaction are other key trait aspects related to conscientiousness: People scoring high in this trait have more intrinsic and extrinsic career success and better job performance; in education they have higher GPAs and increased academic performance; in more general terms, they express greater life satisfaction and higher self-esteem.

Social Networking vs. Conscientiousness?

Though FFT offers conscientiousness as the single most critical health trait, the research compiled by Friedman and Martin makes a case for social networking: "Social relations," they write, "should be the first place to look for improving health and longevity" (*Longevity Project* p. 167). We can agree in part: Extraversion and agreeableness do have health roles to play, too. As Dr. Shealy writes in *Living Bliss* (p. 31): "Over and over," the Longevity Project's participants "emphasized that helping, advising, and caring for others were among the most powerful factors for men and women in leading longer and healthier lives." Of course, we need to consider the quality—and, nowadays, the technology—of interaction. In recent years, social networking websites have dominated the news, but the types of social networking studied over the past eighty years (and reported in Friedman and Martin's book, *Longevity Project*) did not include Facebook, Twitter, Instagram, and other web-based media. Rather, the types of engagement studied by Friedman and Martin stressed "frequency of visiting and communicating with relatives, friends and neighbors," both individually and "in meetings with social or community groups" (p. 160). They included "community service" while depending heavily on "friendships and social contacts," on "intimate and companionate relationships," and on "quality relationships with family and close relatives" (p. 160)—the sorts of relationship in which conscientious individuals thrive.

Perhaps a blog post can count for meaningful interaction. Can it generate the same energy of eye contact while stimulating body and brain together, bathing us in oxytocin and other "feel good" hormones? Even living, breathing phone conversations with friends and relatives seem more capable of activating oxytocin. Now, maybe if you applied Air Bliss prior to blogging, you might at least optimize oxytocin! But our discussion of essential oils must wait ...

Returning to the holistic health metaphor of a wheel, we'll keep conscientiousness at its axle-center and add social networking as an FTT-inspired spoke.

Growing Conscientious.

While we normally think of responsibility, organization, and even conscientiousness as habits of lifestyle, such traits as these have a biological basis. It's the *science* as well as the practice of conscientiousness that we're exploring in this chapter.[3] So, we've arrived at the question lying at the heart of this book: If conscientiousness is so important in our lives, can one become *more* conscientious? Some psychologists take the hardline stance that personality is inborn; in which case, a trait like conscientiousness cannot be changed. Others leave room for some small growth in adulthood. We've already cited evidence from Costa and McCrae, which "suggested very small but consistent

---

3 We've already mentioned *Living Bliss*. Please add that to your reading list, along with the eBook, *30 Days to Self-Health* (Bloomington, IN: Balboa Press, 2018), co-authored by Drs. Shealy and Sorin. We'd also recommend Friedman and Martin's Longevity Project.

Though science-based, the above books aim at a general readership. For more specialist studies, see Brent W. Roberts, et al., "What is Conscientiousness and how can it be assessed?" *Developmental Psychology* 50 (2014): 1315-30, and Richard A. Depue and Paul F. Collins, "Neurobiology of the structure of personality: Dopamine, facilitation of incentive motivation and extraversion," *Behavioral and Brain Sciences* 22 (1999): 491-569.

changes in Neuroticism, Extraversion, and Openness after age 30" (*Personality in Adulthood* p. 155). It's true that our personality traits are relatively stable. It's true, too, that personality has a relatively high heritability rate, with estimates ranging from 41% to as high as 61% heritability. Of the FTT "big five," conscientiousness in particular shows approximately 44% heritability. So, yes, genetics plays a large role in determining our personality traits. Still, a significant portion—over 50%—of personality is impacted by the environment. And this is where epigenetics comes into play. Our genes put us in a certain range of dominant trait characteristics, but the environment and our behavior determine *where we will fall within that range*. So, back to the question at hand: Can one become more conscientious? The answer to this question is—yes!

We should begin by noting that some growth is natural. For most, conscientiousness increases throughout one's life, with the greatest increase in mid-adulthood and older adulthood. Specifically, changes in industriousness, impulse control, reliability, and conventionality are seen in the majority of the population due to aging. Life experiences— stable marriages and stable career paths, for example— can also see increases in levels of conscientiousness. Therapy works, as well: Research has shown that drug rehabilitation treatment and counseling can lead to an increase in conscientiousness. Intense interpersonal therapy for trauma can increase conscientiousness. More recently, it was found that long-term mindfulness training can increase conscientiousness. In the first two cases just mentioned, specific treatments aimed at relieving addictive behaviors and anxiety; in the third case, the training aimed at relaxation in mind and body. In each instance, the change in personality—specifically, the growth in conscientiousness—was a byproduct. That is, the growth was neither conscious nor intentional on the part of those undergoing addiction rehab, trauma therapy, or mindfulness training. From a holistic health perspective, such side-effect growth is not surprising: Positive change in one area leads naturally to positive change in others. But can people consciously, *intentionally* change their conscientiousness level?

Dr. Massey-Abernathy has recently completed two studies where personality was intentionally changed. One study specifically targeted the trait of conscientiousness. In that first study, individuals took part in an eight-week behavioral activation training program. The program included life assessment, goal-creation (starting with small goals and moving up to larger ones), and self-monitoring of activities; throughout the eight-week program, social support was provided and behavioral change rewarded. Participants self-reported more logical thought processing and increased preparedness—both trait aspects of conscientiousness. But that wasn't all. Participants reported that, as their conscientiousness level increased, they experienced an increase in energy and felt fewer limitations in their lives from emotional problems. Here, too, a positive change in one area led naturally to positive changes in others.

In a second study, Dr. Massey-Abernathy and coauthor Dallas N. Robinson allowed participants—116 students enrolled in a psychology course at Missouri State University—to pick any or all of the "big five" factors that they felt needed to change in their lives. Through coaching, she gave simple instructions on how one could change those areas, offering reminders and additional help (if needed) every two weeks for a total of twelve weeks. Participants were asked to track what aspects of their personality they tried to change and why. Again, results showed a change in personality: Students increased their levels of conscientiousness, extraversion, and agreeableness while decreasing neuroticism. The only FFT trait that didn't show change was openness. Again, these trait changes led to changes in physical and emotional health. At the completion of the study, participants reported greater emotional wellbeing and better general health perceptions.[4]

---

4 See Amber R. Massey-Abernathy and Dallas N. Robinson, "Personality Promotion: The Impact of Coaching and Behavioral Activation on Facet Level Personality Change and Health Outcomes," *Current Psychology* 52.2 (June 2019). We quote from the advance copy; the final copy is available at link.springer.com.

The authors observe that "changes in personality facets [relate] to changes in emotional well-being," and that "increased extraversion, increased agreeableness, and decreased neuroticism were related to increased emotional well-being" (p. 11) Similarly, "high extraversion and agreeableness have also been associated with higher life satisfaction," "high stable self-esteem," and "likeability, all of which "can be associated with better emotional well-being. Lower neuroticism is also associated with likeability ... and self-esteem" (p. 11). Their work "also showed physical health impacted by facet change in personality" (p. 11). In their conclusion, Massey-Abernathy and Robinson write:

These studies suggest that facets of personality may be changed, in the direction desired by the individual, through intentional and structured goal setting. The studies also suggest that it may be beneficial in both emotional and physical aspects of one's life to work to change their personality. (p. 11)

Expanding FFT Research. Though psychology has taught us much already, conscientiousness and its trait aspects have social, environmental, interpersonal, physiological, and spiritual components. These and other fields have more to teach us, then. More research needs to be pursued on the IQ average of conscientious individuals, on social and parental influences (e.g., whether parental personalities are formative on a child's level of conscientiousness), on the effects of nutrition and exercise, and on specific tools and techniques that might enhance conscientiousness. We might also ask: Can conscientiousness be increased by means of the following?

Education.
Role models.
Self-Regulation.
Encouragement.
Rewards.
Punishment.
Self-esteem enhancement.
Oxytocin stimulation.
Heart-centered meditation.

We also need to study the neurochemistry of specific personality traits. Do any of the following increase conscientiousness?

Serotonin.

Beta endorphin.

Dopamine.

Oxytocin.

Neurotensin.

Acetylcholine.

We have argued that oxytocin enhancement shows the greatest promise in improving conscientiousness, though we need further clinical/experimental study.

If you're reading this book conscientiously, you'll soon be scoring yourself on the Total Life Stress Assessment, the Self-Rating Depression Scale, and the Shealy-Sorin Anxiety Index. We've got one more self-assessment for you, a Conscientiousness Traits Test (CTT). In order to get a "baseline reading" on your current level of conscientiousness, we ask that you fill out the following honestly—and have your spouse, a close friend, or one of your parents "grade" you by filling out the same questionnaire on your behalf.

Inventorying Conscientiousness.

The FFT-inspired International Personality Item Pool (IPIP) is a self-report assessment tool available online and free of charge.[5] We urge readers to take the full online

_____

5 To take the IPIP inventory, follow this link: http://www.personal.psu.edu/~j5j/IPIP/. See also the IPIP homepage, https://ipip.ori.org/. For

inventory and meditate on its results. The CCT following gives a partial inventory of trait adjectives focused on conscientiousness. In your responses, mark "yes" with a plus sign (+) and "no" with a negative sign (–).

Would you describe yourself as...

Accepting?	( )	Ambitious?	( )
Angry?	( )	Anxiety?	( )
Apathetic?	( )	Awake?	( )
Awesome?	( )	Conscientious?	( )
Cosmic?	( )	Courageous?	( )
Craving?	( )	Critical?	( )
Daydreaming?	( )	Depressed?	( )
Desiring?	( )	Destructive?	( )
Detached (from things you cannot change)? ( )			
Desiring?	( )	Eager?	( )
Enlightened?	( )	Evil?	( )
Extraverted?	( )	Fearful?	( )
Grieving?	( )	Guilty?	( )
Imagining?	( )	Introverted?	( )
Intuitive?	( )	Joyous?	( )
Loving?	( )	Meditative?	( )
Neutral?	( )	Open?	( )
Organized?	( )	Peaceful?	( )

---

a detailed discussion of FFT test design, see Paul T. Costa and Robert R. McCrae, *The NEO Personality Inventory Manual* (Odessa, FL: Psychological Assessment Resources, 1985).

Positive?	( )	Proud?	( )
Reasonable?	( )	Responsible?	( )
Reverent?	( )	Shameful?	( )
Spiritual?	( )	Transcendent?	( )
Willing?	( )		

In a footnote, we give "the typically more conscientious" response.[6] You might compare your results with those given below.

For sixty consecutive days, you'll be asked to practice the big five health essentials (outlined above) and do the Shealy-Sorin Biogenics Self-Regulation System (described below, in Chapter 3). Then, you'll repeat the CCT. If you remain faithful to the Biogenics program, we predict that your CTT scores will improve. And we predict, further, that increased conscientiousness will lead to measurable improvement in health. As reinforcement, you'll be asked to write an essay or two summarizing your experiences and insights. Note that your exploration of conscientiousness requires some

---

6   Though some are neutral (either +/- or -/+) regarding this particular trait, the "more conscientious" responses follow:

Accepting (+); Ambitious (+); Angry (–); Anxiety (–); Apathetic (–); Awake (+); Awesome (+); Conscientious (+); Cosmic (+); Courageous (+); Craving (–); Critical (+/–); Daydreaming (+/–); Depressed (–); Desiring (+); Destructive (–); Detached (from things you cannot change) (+); Desiring (+); Eager (+);Enlightened (+); Evil (–); Extraverted (+); Fearful (–); Grieving (–/+); Guilty (–/+); Imagining (+/–); Introverted (+/–); Intuitive (+); Joyous (+); Loving (+); Meditative (+); Neutral (+/-); Open (+); Organized (+); Peaceful (+); Positive (+); Proud (+); Reasonable (+); Responsible (+); Reverent (+); Shameful (–/+); Spiritual (+); Transcendental (+); Willing (+).

maturity in self-consciousness. Though interrelated, these are not quite the same: Self-consciousness requires mental awareness, alertness, sensitivity, and a healthy capacity for self-reflection and mindfulness. (Within Five-Factor Theory, these are traits commonly associated with openness.)

With respect to health specifically, conscientious people take care over diet, sleep, and exercise; they manage stress; they are mindful and spiritually motivated. Hormonally, they tend to have high levels of dopamine, serotonin, and oxytocin. Adding all these qualities together, we can declare that conscientious people live happier, healthier, longer lives. In contrast, people lacking in conscientiousness live less healthy, less happy, shorter lives. Among their common maladies, people lacking in conscientiousness have higher levels of CRP (that is, C-reactive protein implicated in LDL cholesterol, cardiovascular disease, and acute/ chronic inflammation); they have higher levels of Interleukin-6 (implicated in rheumatoid arthritis and other inflammatory conditions); they may suffer from alexithymia (a subclinical psychiatric disorder marked by social detachment, lack of empathy, and an ability to identify and express one's feelings); they are inclined to addictive and self-destructive behaviors; and, statistically, they have higher rates of suicide.

To conclude this discussion: A list follows of habits, attitudes, traits, and tendencies associated with conscientiousness—and with the lack thereof. Where do you place yourself? Where would you *want* to place yourself?

Conscientious people	People lacking in conscientiousness
are orderly and organized;	are disorganized;
are responsible;	are unreliable; often miss schedules;
are self-disciplined;	lack discipline and motivation;
are competent, confident;	show higher levels of neuroticism;
are achievement-oriented;	lack confidence; fall short of goals;
are positive in attitude;	show higher stress levels;
are more forgiving.	are subject to mood swings/anger.

It's time to write a personal essay. Here's your theme: "Why I am (or am not) optimally conscientious."

3. Self-Diagnosis: The Next Steps

Our readers, we trust, aren't just reading but are *doing* the assessments and protocols described herein. (We'll assume, at least, that that's the case.) So, now that you've inventoried your personality and its dominant traits, we can proceed to an inventory of medical conditions, including your current levels of physical, emotional, and environmental stress. By now, you understand that the fullness and honesty of your responses will reflect your level of conscientiousness. (As we've noted, conscientious health care begins with self-knowledge.) Equally important, you'll understand that that same level of conscientiousness provides a baseline measure of your current overall health. For, holistically, we cannot separate the personality from other aspects of a person's physical-emotional-spiritual wellbeing. More than a state of mind, body, or spirit, conscientious health care is an *activity*: an attitude put into action.

In early years of his private practice, Dr. Shealy administered the Minnesota Multiphasic Personality Inventory (MMPI) to clients; later, he used the California Psychological Inventory (CPI). Currently, clients of the Shealy-Sorin Wellness Institute are given the Total Life Stress Test (TLS), based (with permission from Dr. T. H. Holmes) on the Holmes-Rahe Social Readjustment Rating Scale (SRRS).[7]

First, we're going to take the SRRS and calculate your total score. We'll then convert that score into a TLS number-equivalent—but we'll explain that later. Here's the SRRS:

Mark the life events listed below that you have experienced during the past 12 months:

Death of spouse	100_____
Divorce	73_____
Marital separation	65_____
Jail time	63_____

---

7   See, e.g., T. H. Holmes and R. H. Rahe, "The social readjustment rating scale," *Journal of Psychosomatic Research* 11 (1967): 213-18.

Death of close family member	63_____
Personal injury or illness	53_____
Marriage	50_____
Fired at work	47_____
Marital reconciliation	45_____
Retirement	45_____
Change in health of family member	44_____
Pregnancy	40_____
Sexual difficulties	39_____
Gain of new family member	39_____
Business readjustment	39_____
Change in financial state	38_____
Death of close friend	37_____
Change to different line of work	36_____
Change in number of arguments with spouse	35_____
Mortgage over $200,000	31_____
Foreclosure of mortgage or loan	30_____
Change in responsibilities at work	29_____
Son or daughter leaving home	29_____
Trouble with in-laws	29_____
Outstanding personal achievement	28_____
Spouse begin or stop work	26_____
Begin or end school	25_____
Change in living conditions	24_____
Revision of personal habits	23_____
Trouble with boss	20_____
Change in work hours or conditions	20_____
Change in residence	20_____

Change in schools	19_____
Change in recreation	19_____
Change in church activities	18_____
Change in social activities	17_____
Mortgage or loan less than $200,000	16_____
Change in sleeping habits	15_____
Change in eating habits	15_____
Vacation, especially if away from home	13_____
Christmas, or other major holiday stress	12_____
Minor violations of the law	11_____

YOUR TOTAL SRRS SCORE _____

Now, we're going to convert your total score on Holmes-Rahe Social Readjustment Rating Scale to its equivalent on the Shealy-Sorin Total Life Stress Test (TLS). Here's the conversion table:

SRRS less than 60:	TLS 0	SRRS less than 110:	TLS 1
SRRS less than 160:	TLS 2	SRRS less than 170:	TLS 3
SRRS less than 180:	TLS 4	SRRS less than 190:	TLS 5
SRRS less than 200:	TLS 6	SRRS less than 210:	TLS 7
SRRS less than 220:	TLS 8	SRRS less than 230:	TLS 9
SRRS less than 240:	TLS 10	SRRS less than 250:	TLS 11
SRRS less than 260:	TLS 11	SRRS less than 265:	TLS 12
SRRS less than 270:	TLS 13	SRRS less than 275:	TLS 14
SRRS less than 280:	TLS 15	SRRS less than 285:	TLS 16
SRRS less than 290:	TLS 17	SRRS less than 295:	TLS 18
SRRS less than 300:	TLS 19	SRRS less than 305:	TLS 20

And so on, adding one TLS point per five additional SRRS points. You're going to add thus converted score to the TLS subtotal F, below. And now for the Shealy-Sorin Total Life Stress Test. Please respond to it conscientiously.

TOTAL LIFE STRESS TEST

Name:_____

Date: _____

Record your stress points on the lines in the right-hand margin and indicate subtotals in the boxes at the end of each section. Then add your subtotals to determine your total score.

A. DIETARY STRESS

Average Daily Sugar Consumption

Sugar added to food or drink

1 point per 5 tsp _____

Sweet Roll, piece of pie/ cake, brownie, other dessert

1 point each _____

Coke or can of pop; candy bar

2 points each _____

Banana Split, commercial milk shake, sundae, etc.

5 points each _____

White flour (white bread, spaghetti, etc.)

5 points _____

Average Daily Salt Consumption

Little or no "added" salt

0 points _____

Few salty foods (pretzels, potato chips, etc.)

0 points _____

Moderate "added" salt and/ or salty foods

at least once per day   *3 points* _____

Heavy salt user, regularly (use of "table salt" and/or salty

foods at least twice per day)   *10 points* _____

Average Daily Caffeine Consumption

Coffee

½ point each cup _____

Tea

½ point each cup _____

Cola drink or Mountain Dew

1 point each cup _____

2 Anacin or APC tabs

½ point per dose _____

Caffeine Benzoate tablets (NoDoz, Vivrin, etc.)

2 points each _____

Average Weekly Eating Out

2-4 times per week

3 points _____

5-10 times per week

6 points _____

More than 10 times per week

10 points _____

  DIETARY SUBTOTAL A _____

B. ENVIRONMENTAL STRESS
Drinking Water

Chlorinated only

*1 point*_____

Chlorinated and fluoridated

*2 points*_____

Soil and Air Pollution

Live within 10 miles of city of 500,000 or more

*10 points*_____

Live within 10 miles of city of 250,000 or more

*5 points*_____

Live within 10 miles of city of 50,000 or more

*2 points*_____

Live in the country but use pesticides, herbicides and/or

chemical fertilizer   *10 points*_____

Soil and Air Pollution

Exposed to cigarette smoke of someone else

more than 1 hour per day

*5 points*_____

Television Watched

For each hour over 1 per day

*½ point*_____

    ENVIRONMENTAL SUBTOTAL B_____

C. CHEMICAL STRESS

Drugs (any amount of usage)

Antidepressants

*1 point*_____

Tranquilizers

*3 points*_____

Sleeping pills

3 points_____

Narcotics

5 points_____

Other pain relievers

3 points_____

Nicotine

3-10 cigarettes per day

5 points_____

11-20 cigarettes per day

15 points_____

21-30 cigarettes per day

20 points_____

31-40 cigarettes per day

35 points_____

Over 40 cigarettes per day

40 points_____

Cigar(s) per day

1 point each_____

Pipeful(s) of tobacco per day

1 point each_____

Chewing tobacco – "chews" per day

1 point each_____

Average Daily Alcohol Consumption 1 oz. whiskey, gin,

vodka, etc.   *2 points each_____*

8 oz. beer

2 points each_____

4-6 oz. glass of wine

2 points each_____

CHEMICAL SUBTOTAL C_____

D. PHYSICAL STRESS
Weight

Underweight more than 10 lbs.

5 points_____

10-15 lbs. overweight

5 points_____

16-25 lbs. overweight

10 points_____

26-40 lbs. overweight

25 points_____

More than 40 lbs. overweight

40 points_____

Activity

Adequate exercise,8 3 days or more per week

0 points_____

Some physical exercise, 1 or 2 days per week

15 points_____

No regular Exercise

40 points_____

Work Stress

Sit most of the day

3 points_____

Industrial/ factory worker

3 points_____

---

8 "Adequate" means doubling heartbeat and/or sweating a minimum of 30 minutes per session.

Overnight travel more than once a week

5 points_____

Work more than 50 hours per week

2 points per hour Over 50_____

Work Varying shifts

10 points_____

Work night shifts

5 points _____

PHYSICAL SUBTOTAL D_____

E. EMOTIONAL STRESS

Sleep

Less than 7 hours per night

3 points_____

Usually 7 to 8 hours per night

0 points _____

More than 8 hours per night

2 points _____

Relaxation

Relax only during sleep

10 points_____

Relax or mediate at least 20 minutes per day

0 points_____

Frustration at work

Enjoy Work

0 points _____

Mildly frustrated by job

1 point _____

Moderately frustrated by job

3 points _____

Very frustrated by job

5 points _____

Marital Status

Married, happily

0 points _____

Married, moderately unhappy

2 points _____

Married, very unhappy

5 points _____

Unmarried man over 30

5 points _____

Unmarried woman over 30

2 points _____

Usual Mood

Happy, well-adjusted

0 points _____

Moderately angry depressed or frustrated

10 points _____

Very angry, depressed or frustrated

20 points _____

Any Other Major Stress Not Mentioned Above

You Judge Intensity (Specify):

10 to 40 points _____

EMOTIONAL SUBTOTAL E _____

F. YOUR CONVERTED SRRS SCORE

SUBTOTAL F _____

Add A _____ + B _____ + C _____ + D _____ + E _____ + F _____ = YOUR PERSONAL STRESS ASSESSMENT SCORE

If your total score is over 50, make a concerted effort to reduce your stress!

Here's another self-evaluation questionnaire used at the Shealy-Sorin Wellness Institute. This inventory aims at the variety of symptoms—physical, emotional, behavioral—present in a client's current illness or condition.

Symptom Index

Name: _____

Date: _____

When people are chronically ill, they often have other symptoms. Do you have any of the following?

PLEASE CHECK ONLY THOSE THAT YOU HAVE NOW OR HAVE HAD WITH YOUR CURRENT ILLNESS.

_____ Depressed mood.

_____ Loss of interest or pleasure in things you used to enjoy.

_____ Significant weight change (loss or gain).

_____ Frequent eating between meals.

_____ Insomnia.

_____ Snoring.

_____ Sleep walking.

_____ Hypersomnia.

_____ Agitation.

_____ Sluggishness, slow to function.

_____ Fatigue, low energy, feeling tired all of the time.

_____ Feelings of worthlessness or guilt.

_____ Difficulty concentrating, thinking, and remembering.

_____ Indecisiveness.

_____ Recurrent thoughts of death or suicide.

_____ Suicide attempts.

_____ Nervous exhaustion.

_____ Worrying excessively or being anxious.

_____ Frequent crying.

_____ Being extremely shy or sensitive.

_____ Lumps or swelling in your neck.

_____ Blurring of vision.

_____ Seeing double.

_____ Seeing colored halos around lights.

_____ Pains or itching around the eyes.

_____ Excess blinking or watering of the eyes.

_____ Loss of vision.

_____ Difficulty hearing.

_____ Earache.

_____ Running ear.

_____ Buzzing or other noises in the ears.

_____ Motion sickness.

_____ Teeth or gum problems.

_____ Sore or sensitive tongue.

_____ Change in sense of taste.

_____ Nose stuffed up.

_____ Runny nose.

_____ Sneezing spells.

_____ Frequent head colds.

_____ Bleeding from the nose.

_____ Sore throat even without cold.

_____ Enlarged tonsils.

_____ Hoarse voice even without cold.

_____ Difficulty or pain in swallowing.

_____ Wheezing or difficulty breathing.

_____ Coughing spells.

_____ Coughing up a lot of phlegm.

_____ Coughing up blood.

_____ Chest colds more than once a month.

_____ High blood pressure.

_____ Low blood pressure.

_____ Heart trouble.

_____ Thumping or racing heart.

_____ Pain or tightness in the chest.

_____ Shortness of breath.

_____ Heartburn.

_____ Feeling bloated.

_____ Excess belching.

_____ Discomfort in the pit of your stomach.

_____ Nausea.

_____ Vomiting blood.

_____ Peptic ulcer.

_____ Change in appetite.

_____ Digestive problems.

_____ Excess hunger.

_____ Getting up frequently at night to urinate.

_____ Urinating more than 5-6 times a day.

_____ Unable to control your urine.

_____ Burning or pains when you urinate.

_____ Black, brown, or bloody urine.

_____ Difficulty starting your urine.

_____ Constant urge to urinate.

_____ Constipation.

_____ Diarrhea.

_____ Black or bloody bowel movement.

_____ Grey bowel movement.

_____ Pain when you move your bowels.

_____ Bleeding from your rectum.

_____ Stomach pains which double you up.

_____ Frequent stomach trouble.

_____ Intestinal worms.

_____ Hemorrhoids.

_____ Yellow jaundice.

_____ Biting your nails.

_____ Stuttering or stammering.

_____ Any kind of problem with your genital or sexual organs.

_____ Sexual problems.

_____ Hernia or rupture.

_____ Kidney or bladder disease.

_____ Stiff or Painful muscles or joints.

_____ Swelling joints.

_____ Pain in your back or shoulders.

_____ Painful feet.

_____ Swelling in your armpits or groin.

_____ Trouble with swollen feet or ankles.

_____ Cramps in your legs at night or with walking.

_____ Itching or burning skin.

_____ Rash or pimples.

_____ Excess bleeding from a small cut.

_____ Easy burning skin.

_____ Dizziness or light headedness.

_____ Feeling faint or fainting.

_____ Numbness in any part of your body.

_____ Cold hands or feet even in hot water.

_____ Paralysis.

_____ Blacking out.

_____ Fits, convulsions, or epilepsy.

_____ Change in your handwriting.

_____ Tendency to shake or tremble.

_____ Tendency to be too hot or too cold.

_____ Sweating more than usual.

_____ Hot flashes.

_____ Being short of breath with minimal effort.

_____ Failure to get adequate exercise.

_____ Being overweight.

_____ Being underweight.

_____ Having lost more than half of your teeth.

_____ Bleeding gums.

_____ Badly coated tongue.

_____ A lot of small accident or injuries.

_____ Varicose veins.

_____ Headaches.

_____ Other aches and pains.

_____ Feeling pessimistic or hopeless.

_____ Have had any kind of surgery within
the past year.

_____ Being upset easily by criticism.

_____ Having little annoyances get on your nerves
and make you angry.

_____ Getting angry easily.

_____ Getting nervous around strangers.

_____ Feeling lonely.

_____ Having difficulty relaxing.

_____ Being troubled by frightening dreams
or thoughts.

_____ Being disturbed by work or family problems.

_____ Wishing that you could get psychological or
psychiatric help.

_____ Being tense or jittery.

_____ Being easily upset.

_____ Being in low spirits.

_____ Being in very low spirits.

_____ Believing that your life is out of your hands
and controlled by external forces.

_____ Feeling that life is empty, filled with despair.

_____ Having no goals or aims at all.

_____ Having failed to make progress towards your life goals.

_____ Feeling that you are completely bound by factors outside yourself.

_____ Feeling sad, blue, or down in the dumps.

_____ Feeling slowed down or restless and unable to sit still.

_____ Frequent illness.

_____ Being confined to bed by illness.

For men only:

_____ Having a urine stream that's very weak or very slow.

_____ Having prostate trouble.

_____ Having unusual burning or discharge from your penis.

_____ Having swelling or lumps in your testicles.

_____ Having your testicles painful.

_____ Having trouble getting erections (getting hard).

For women only:

_____ Having trouble with your menstrual period.

_____ Bleeding between your periods.

_____ Having heavy bleeding with your periods.

_____ Getting bloated or irritable before your periods.

_____ Taking birth control pills (in the last year).

_____ Having lumps in your breasts.

_____ Having excess discharge from your vagina.
_____ Feeling weak or sick with your periods.
_____ Having to lie down when your periods start.
_____ Feeling tense and jumpy with your periods.
_____ Having constant hot flashes and sweats.
_____ Have had a hysterectomy or on
hormonal replacement.

If you've checked more than twenty symptoms, then it's likely that overall stress is affecting your physiology and that "unfinished business" (emotional, relational, spiritual) is hindering your health! Ultimately, your number one key to optimizing health is to reduce all stress and its symptoms. Once you are physically, emotionally, and spiritually balanced, you're ready to develop your optimal health.

The Zung Self-Rating Depression Scale (SDS) offers a further useful tool in self-diagnosis.[9] Each of its statements is weighted by duration of mood or behavior (e.g., you feel sad "none or little of the time," "some of the time," "good part of the time," or "most or all of the time," with a numeric value assigned to each). Once again, it's time to be brutally honest with yourself. By circling the numbers that best describe you, fill out the following to see whether you're depressed.

---

9 See W. W. Zung, "A Self-Rating Depression Scale," *Archives of General Psychiatry,* January 12, 1965, pp. 63-70.

Name:			None or a Little of the Time	Some of the Time	Good Part of the Time	Most or All of the Time
Age:	Sex:	Date:				
1. I FEEL DOWN-HEARTED, BLUE AND SAD.			1	2	3	4
2. MORNING IS WHEN I FEEL THE BEST.			4	3	2	1
3. I HAVE CRYING SPELLS OR FEEL LIKE IT.			1	2	3	4
4. I HAVE TROUBLE SLEEPING THROUGH. THE NIGHT.			1	2	3	4
5. I EAT AS MUCH AS I USED TO.			4	3	2	1
6. I ENJOY LOOKING AT, TALKING TO AND BEING WITH ATTRACTIVE WOMEN/MEN.			4	3	2	1
7. I NOTICE THAT I AM LOSING WEIGHT.			1	2	3	4
8. I HAVE TROUBLE WITH CONSTIPATION.			1	2	3	4
9. MY HEART BEATS FASTER THAN USUAL.			1	2	3	4
10. I GET TIRED FOR NO REASON.			1	2	3	4
11. MY MIND IS AS CLEAR AS IT USED TO BE.			4	3	2	1
12. I FIND IT EASY TO DO THE THINGS I USED TO BE.			4	3	2	1
13. I AM RESTLESS AND CAN'T KEEP STILL.			1	2	3	4
14. I FEEL HOPEFULE ABOUT THE FUTURE.			4	3	2	1
15. I AM MORE IRRITABLE THAN USUAL.			1	2	3	4
16. I FIND IT EASY TO MAKE DECISIONS.			4	3	2	1
17. I FEEL THAT I AM USEFUL AND NEEDED.			4	3	2	1
18. MY LIFE IS PRETTY FULL.			4	3	2	1
19. I FEEL THAT OTHERS WOULD BE BETTER OFF IF I WERE DEAD.			1	2	3	4
20. I STILL ENJOY THE THINGS I USED TO DO.			4	3	2	1

SDS RAW SCORE_____

If your raw score is forty or above, then the Depression Scale gives strong evidence that you're clinically depressed. If your score lies between thirty and thirty-nine, then you'd be subclinically depressed (*and that still ain't good*).

If you're subject to depression, there's a fifty-fifty chance that you experience anxiety as well. As Kathleen Smith notes, "there is some overlap" between the two: "Sleep problems, trouble concentrating, and fatigue are all symptoms of both anxiety and depression. Irritability may also manifest in forms of anxiety or depression (in place of low mood)."[10] At the Wellness Institute, we rely on a self-rating scale similar to the numeric rating scale (NRS) of pain:

Shealy-Sorin Anxiety Index.

Fear, worry, and anxiety are the major reactions to stress. For the following statements, circle the number that reflects your anxiety level:

Anxiety causes me insomnia.

1 - 2 - 3 - 4 - 5 - 6 - 7 - 8 - 9 - 10

Anxiety prevents me from being happy.

1 - 2 - 3 - 4 - 5 - 6 - 7 - 8 - 9 - 10

Anxiety interferes with my work.

1 - 2 - 3 - 4 - 5 - 6 - 7 - 8 - 9 - 10

I have health problems.

1 - 2 - 3 - 4 - 5 - 6 - 7 - 8 - 9 - 10

Anxiety interferes with my social life.

1 - 2 - 3 - 4 - 5 - 6 - 7 - 8 - 9 - 10

My greatest anxiety is my family.

1 - 2 - 3 - 4 - 5 - 6 - 7 - 8 - 9 - 10

My greatest anxiety is financial.

1 - 2 - 3 - 4 - 5 - 6 - 7 - 8 - 9 - 10

My overall level of anxiety:

1 - 2 - 3 - 4 - 5 - 6 - 7 - 8 - 9 - 10

---

10   Kathleen Smith, "Anxiety vs. Depression: How to Tell the Difference," *PsyCom* (https://www.psycom.net/anxiety-depression-difference), accessed 24 December 2019.

Add all eight NRS responses. If the number reaches sixty or above, *then you, sir (or madam), have severe anxiety!*

Each of these inventories includes questions about sleep and sleep disturbance. There's a good reason for that. Among the five health essentials, we call for "seven or eight hours" of sleep every night. Actually, seven hours is the minimum for optimal health; eight should be our goal. And a good night's sleep has its cascade effect on health. People who sleep well tend to follow the commonsense maxim, "early to bed, early to rise ..." There's a good reason for that, too. Our bodies have circadian rhythms—sleep cycles—when melatonin is produced maximally. Melatonin induces sleep: It's the body's natural sleep hormone, manufactured by the pineal gland. It shouldn't surprise that people who sleep well wake up refreshed and ready for the day. These "morning people" are the envy of those who stay up late, have trouble falling asleep, and tend to wake up late—and irritable, and still tired. Here's the point: Sleep patterns are reflective of personality type, and conscientiousness is the single biggest predictor of diurnal preference.[11]

Morning-preference individuals show a strong correlation between beginning-and-ending sleep time and optimal melatonin production.[12] Higher serotonin levels were

---

11   See Alexandra L. Hogben et al., "Conscientiousness predicts diurnal preference," *Chronobiology International* 24.6 (February 2007): 1249-54.

12   Xianchen Liu et al., "Diurnal preferences, sleep habits, circadian sleep propensity and melatonin rhythm in healthy human subjects," *Neuroscience Letters* 280.3 (February 2000):199-202.

found in morning people, whereas evening-preference people (adolescents especially) showed lower serotonin levels, as well as higher levels of neuroticism, aggression, and anti-social behaviors.[13] Morning people tend to be more stable—the opposite of neuroticism within the FFT model. All of which leads us to restate our thesis: Virtually all risky health-related behaviors show a lack of conscientiousness, while beneficial health-related behaviors abound in conscientiousness.[14]

4. After Diagnosis: "What next?"

By now, it's obvious that conscientiousness affects the whole person—body, mind, and spirit. More than habit and attitude, conscientiousness has genetic and environmental components; its expressions are emotional and physiological—indeed, neurochemical and hormonal. It affects our love life, our work life, our prayer life. Of necessity, then, a holistic approach to health care must

---

13 Colin G. DeYoung et al., "Morning people are stable people: Circadian rhythm and the higher-order factors of the Big Five," *Personality and Individual Differences* 43 (2007): 267-2766. As I write in *Living Bliss*, "conscientious people do more to protect their health. They engage in fewer risky activities. They're less likely to smoke, less likely to drink excessively, less likely to do drugs, and less likely to drive too fast. Conscientious people tend to take more safety precautions and are more likely to wear seat belts" (p. 23).

Howard S. Friedman and Leslie L. Martin—co-authors of *The Longevity Project*—observe that serotonin is necessary "to regulate many health-relevant processes throughout the body, including how much you eat and how well you sleep" (*Living Bliss*, p. 23). Through our own research, we've noted that individuals with low serotonin levels are more impulsive and that low serotonin is a major foundation of depression.

14 See Tim Bogg and Brent W. Roberts, "Conscientiousness and health-related behaviors: A meta-analysis of the leading behavioral contributors to mortality," *Psychological Bulletin* 130 (2004): 887-919.

approach conscientiousness holistically, as well. When one makes a habit of *acting* conscientiously, one learns *to think* conscientiously and reaps the blissful benefits—physiological, hormonal, emotional, spiritual—accruing thereto. Concomitantly, a habit *of thinking* conscientiously leads one *to act* conscientiously, which yields those same blissful benefits. Let's go further: If one can learn *to speak* conscientiously, then one can learn *to think* conscientiously, which will lead one *to act* conscientiously. Further still, one can learn *to listen* to another's calming words, allowing them soft, whispering entry into one's own mind and imagination: Providing instructions in relaxation, these words can be translated into one's own thoughtful response *and put into action,* making them habitual. Through what's left of this chapter, we'll be exploring ways to reduce stress and enhance health energetically. Rejecting knife-and-pill allopathy, we'll introduce readers to modalities of autogenic training, scalar wave, and hormonal balancing through brainwave frequency.

Autogenic training(AT)—the power of verbal suggestion—is the means by which one learns to listen, speak, think, and act habitually *in bliss,* as described above. Akin to self-hypnosis, AT was pioneered by German psychiatrist, Johannes Heinrich Shultz (1884-1970).[15] It is

---

15 Since 1928, Dr. Shultz's autogenic training has had more published proof than any other relaxation technique, with 27,000 scholarly references to date. See N. Kanji, "Autogenic Training," *Complementary Therapies in Medicine* 5 (1997): 162–167. See also Friedhelm Stetter and Sirko Kupper, "Autogenic training: A meta-analysis of clinical outcome studies," *Applied Psychophysiology and Biofeedback* 27 (2002): 45–98.

by means of AT that our sixty-day Biogenics course in conscientious health care proceeds.

Autogenic Training (Basic Schultz). Available at our Wellness Institute,[16] this eighteen-minute audio recording is the foundation of the Shealy-Sorin Biogenics Self-Regulation System. It makes use of Dr. Schultz's original instructions (hence the name, "Basic Schultz"), though these have been updated for use in the Biogenics system. A series of seven affirmations are repeated slowly, to which the trainee (reclining comfortably while wearing headphones) gives "passive concentration":

> My arms and legs are heavy and warm.
> My heartbeat is calm and regular.
> My breathing is free and easy.
> My abdomen is warm.
> My forehead is cool.
> My mind is quiet and still.
> I am at peace.

There's a paradox in the phrase, "passive concentration." Even as the trainee focuses on feelings of warmth, coolness, and calmness, these feelings are not compelled: Rather than "willed,"

16   A free mp3 of this most essential Biogenics exercise may be found in the Sound/Biogenics section of the Shealy-Sorin Wellness website (www. ShealyWellness.com).

they are "allowed to happen," through the mental-imaginative power of suggestion.

AT is a proven relaxation technique and, when practiced twice daily for a minimum of three months, it has an 85% success rate in retraining/resetting the central and autonomic nervous systems. More than stress management, AT can help with a number of conditions:

- Anxiety, depression, and other mental health aspects.
- Hypertension, diabetes, and other metabolic aspects.
- Pain management, including both chronic and acute pain.
- Problems with sleep, muscle tension, and relaxation.

In place of antidepressants and anti-anxiety medication, we preach autogenic training, among other energy-based CAM therapies.

In 1977, Dr. Shealy was living in La Crosse, Wisconsin, where he had opened his first private practice in alternative medicine—a new field at the time. He was already using AT, both in his practice and in experimental studies. Back then, the football team at the University of Wisconsin-La Crosse was stumbling. So he offered to teach AT to the team. The year before, they were at the bottom of their league; during that year of training, the UWL Eagles were league co-champions. In basketball, the UWL Lady Eagles were next. Half of the team—the "control group"—just practiced; the other half used a special AT and guided imagery tape that Dr. Shealy had recorded for them. The women athletes who used the AT tape were 80% more successful at free throws than those who did not.

Dr. Shealy has continued to study AT and its effects on various conditions in various settings. In a recent study of the effectiveness of an herbal preparation on hypertension, 30% of patients failed to improve with the herb alone. Within ten minutes, AT brought the blood pressure of twelve of fourteen patients down to normal; in follow-up tests, these patients continued their improvement. Using an mp3 recording of AT, one of the Wellness Institute's doctoral students helped caregivers of terminally-ill patients reduce their stress and symptoms at a statistically-significant level. Another doctoral student used an mp3 recording to reduce symptoms significantly in patients with fibromyalgia, one of the most difficult of chronic pain conditions. AT has proven highly successful in helping patients with anxiety, depression, and migraine—all disorders in which oxytocin is low.

AT has helped students improve academically. It's helped business specialists improve performance. It's helped young and old alike. (Cognitively and emotionally, children ought to start training in AT age five!) It doesn't always work, but can you guess why? It's typically not a failure of technique, but rather *of conscientiousness*: Some 80% of patients fail to use AT twice daily as recommended, and many won't use it even once. (How can it work if the trainee won't follow directions?)

Brainwaves and Personality.

As noted, conscientious individuals tend to live long, healthy, happy lives. They're good at what they do. They're good learners, often blessed with a strong memory and imagination; their drive to succeed is sustained by powers of self-discipline and self-control. And one reason they're driven to succeed is the sheer pleasure it gives, not just in the achievement but in the work activity itself. (In effect, they "*are* happy" because they "*do* happy.") They thrive off of the feelings that peak performance and creativity produce—feelings of being "in the zone," when EEG activity is in the Gamma range. Brainwaves are synchronized electronic wave-pulses: They're the means by which neuron clusters communicate with each other. And brain activity is measured by Hertz (Hz) frequency—that is, by speed of oscillation—using an electroencephalogram (EEG). That feeling of being "in the zone" is no mere metaphor: It's a marker of Gamma activity, when brainwaves oscillate in the 40 Hz range or higher. In this range, the individual experiences optimal memory and creativity, improved sensory perception, and greater happiness overall. By contrast, depressed and anxious individuals experience little Gamma wave activity, which is also largely absent in every physical and emotional disease.[17]

Mainstream practitioners talk too often of medication and too rarely of brain activity. Gamma waves, as we've said, are nature's own best antidepressant, creating feelings of "blessedness," bliss, and even ecstasy. Buddhist monks and Celestine nuns produce Gamma waves during meditation. Feelings of love and compassion are also tied to increased Gamma activity. These same emotions are marked by increased production of endorphins, vasopressin and anandamide—all mood-positive neurochemicals.

The fact is that healthy, happy individuals have a broad variability in EEG activity. Healthy individuals when alert and attentive tend to have EEG activity between 14 and 24 Hz, the lower (or "happy") Beta frequency. When they're stressed or anxious, their EEG tends to move into upper Beta frequency, 25 to 30 Hz. When they relax, their EEG activity tends to move into Alpha frequency, 8 to 12 Hz, marked by increased serotonin production. Even deeper relaxation leads to Theta frequency, 4 to 7 Hz, an EEG activity associated with meditation and the dreamy hypnogogic state of near-sleep. As they drift to sleep, their EEG activity

---

17 A. Akpinar, G. B. Yaman, A. Demirdas, and S. Onai, "Possible role of adrenomedullin and nitric oxide in major depression," *Progress in Neuro-Psychopharmacology and Biological Psychiatry* 46 (2013): 120-125.

moves into Delta frequency, 1 to 3 Hz. In each case, the healthy brain shows consistency and symmetry in its brainwave activity. By contrast, depressed and anxious individuals show frontal EEG asymmetry.[18]

Introducing the Shealy-Sorin Gamma PEMF.

Forgive this biochemistry lesson, but every cell in a healthy body has a -70 millivolt (mV) bioelectric charge. When the cell is overstressed, its charge may drop to -50 mV. The single best way to return cells to their normal -70 mV charge is the Gamma PEMF.

Success of the Gamma PEMF brings us to a core insight of energy medicine: Organic life would cease without electromagnetic exchanges at the cellular level. For the body takes its energy from the highly reactive, "high energy" nucleotide, adenosine triphosphate (ATP). As the "universal energy currency for life," ATP stores electrical energy in its three phosphate bonds and releases energy when hydrolyzed into adenosine diphosphate (ADP). Basic biochemistry textbooks describe the Krebs Cycle, glycolysis, and the processes of cellular respiration; yet cellular respiration is merely the most obvious, most observable aspect of "the body electric," as American poet, Walt Whitman (1819-1892), describes the living human creature.

---

18 See R. Thibodeau, R. S. Jorgensen, and S. Kim, "Depression, anxiety, and resting frontal EEG asymmetry: A meta-analytic review," *Journal of Abnormal Psychology* 115.4 (2006): 715-29.

Note the connections between "state of health" and "state of mind" (though "*activity* of mind"—and "*of brain*"— hits closer to home). The Biogenics System achieves healthy EEG activity energetically through the Gamma PEMF machine. Clinical studies performed for the Shealy-Sorin Wellness Institute offer convincing proof that increased Gamma activity can reduce the cravings of opiate addicts in rehab treatment, at the same time increasing their levels of conscientiousness. And it has the potential to improve cognition, perhaps even raising IQ.[19] Revolutionary in its implications/applications, the Gamma PEMF makes a mighty contribution to 21st century holistic health care.

Spirituality and Scalar Energy.

In an FFT-based study of faith traditions (Buddhism, Catholicism, Judaism, Islam, and Protestantism),[20] B. Johnstone et al. found that "better mental health is significantly related to increased spirituality," which correlates positively "with positive personality traits (i.e., extraversion) and negatively with negative

19 E. Santarnecchi, T. Muller, A. Sarkar, N. R. Polizzoto, A. Rossi, and Cohen Kadosh, "Individual differences and specificity of prefrontal Gamma frequency-tACS on fluid intelligence capabilities," *Science Direct* 75 (2016): 33-43.

20 B. Johnstone, D. P. Yoon, D. Cohen, L. H. Schopp, et al., "Relationships among spirituality, religious practices, personality factors, and health for five different faith traditions," *Journal of Religion and Health* 51.4 (2012): 1017-41.

personality traits (i.e., neuroticism)" (p. 1017). For each faith studied, "the presence of positive and absence of negative personality traits are primary predictors of positive health (and primarily mental health)" (p. 1017). Spirituality, thus, is "a characterological aspect of personality" directly conducive of health (Johnstone, p. 1017). As an FFT trait aspect, spirituality is often paired with religiosity, though distinctions can be made: Religiousness, as Corinna E. Löckenhoff and Paul T. Costa note,[21] "encompasses both a specific belief system and a set of behaviors (e.g., prayer, church attendance)," whereas *spirituality* "typically refers to subjective, non-church-centered experiences of the transcendent which imbue everyday life with a sense of deeper meaning" (p. 1411). We're perfectly content to follow Löckenhoff and Costa in pairing the terms, though their own study identifies religiosity "primarily ... with High Conscientiousness and Agreeableness" and spirituality "with high Openness" (Löckenhoff and Costa, p. 1412). Still, their thesis—to which we give hearty agreement—is that "spirituality/religiousness (S/R) have emerged as important predictors of sustained well-being in the face of adversity" (p. 1411). In the midst of severe physical illness, S/R faith preserves a high level of mental health, increasing one's resilience to life's stresses (Löckenhoff and Costa, p. 1411).

---

21 Corinna E. Löckenhoff and Paul T. Costa, "Five-Factor Model Personality Traits, Spirituality/Religiousness, and Mental Health among People Living With HIV," *Journal of Personality* 77.5 (2009): 1411-36.

We want to carry these FFT studies a step further: More than resilience in the face of illness, we look to faith as a means of active healing. Dr. Shealy tells a story in this regard. In 1972, he was introduced to Olga Worrall (1908-1985), Director of the New Life Clinic at Mt. Washington United Methodist Church in Baltimore; she was also the most scientifically-studied healer in history, having healed thousands—many of them physicians and scientists, who took keen interest in her abilities. After witnessing a church service in which she laid hands on some three hundred people, Dr. Shealy was invited into a private healing session between Olga and another visitor. In this private session, he witnessed the most awful breast cancer he had ever seen: a huge, black, necrotic mass. One month later this same woman, a professor of English, reported that her cancer was gone.

Though no skeptic himself, Dr. Shealy sought documentary evidence of Olga's healing powers: These, he believed, would come from the physicians who had treated the patients Olga had healed and could give "before and after" testimony of results. From Olga herself, he received one hundred letters from patients who had written to her, saying they had been healed. He wrote to them all, requesting and receiving permission to write their physicians for medical proof of their healing. Only eleven physicians replied.[22] (Do you, too, wonder why?)

22 But there were more to come. Growing fast lifetime friends with Dr. Shealy, Olga Worrall bequeathed him much of her memorabilia (*Living Bliss* p. 140), including 15,000 letters from her healed patients.
For an account of Olga's spiritual journey together with her husband,

In 1977, Olga came to Dr. Shealy's clinic, where she joined Dr. Elmer Green (1917-2017), famed American physicist and pioneer of biofeedback, in an experiment on "remote healing." Though known for her healing hands, she could heal by mental intention, as well. So, while Dr. Green made EEG recordings of Olga, Dr. Shealy recorded EEGs for twelve different patients whom she worked on, one at a time in different rooms. In each case, there was an instant change in the patient's EEG when Olga sent healing thoughts. Over the years, Dr. Shealy has repeated this experiment, documenting 116 cases of eighteen different healers instantly changing another person's EEG—and doing so from distances up to one thousand miles away.

There's another, more traditional term for remote healing and mental intention: You can call it, simply, *prayer*. That's what Olga and her husband Ambrose practiced at Mt. Washington United Methodist Church. But Western logic has a problem with spiritual healing. Even strongly religious individuals tend to divorce matter from spirit: For many, if a physical healing cannot be explained in physical terms, then it's either a miracle or a hoax. (And since many don't believe in miracles, that leaves only the latter as explanation.) Eastern traditions have long known of this generalized and universally-accessible "life force." In Chinese medicine, it's called *qi*, in Indian Ayurvedic medicine, *prana*. So we must look to holism to heal the mind/body matter/spirit dualism infecting Western

Ambrose Worrall, see *The Gift of Healing: A Personal Story of Spiritual Therapy* (Columbus, OH: Ariel Press, 1985).

thought. And there is, indeed, a physical explanation for this seemingly spiritual/metaphysical phenomenon: It's called scalar wave energy.

The phenomenal beauty of the Universe as we know it and its unlimited power are perhaps best understood through this concept, derived from quantum physics. All "empty space" throughout the Universe is filled with scalar energy. In that infinite scalar field, within a space the size of a mere helium molecule, there's energy sufficient to boil all the Earth's oceans! That's an awesome power, one invoking the world-creating/world-destroying potency of God.

Introducing scalar wave therapy. The Shealy-Sorin sapphire-enhanced scalar machine projects zero-point energy through a crystalline sheet of crushed sapphire. Exposure to scalar energy significantly reduces adrenomedullin, the most important biochemical marker of stress. (Sadly, allopathic practitioners never think to test for adrenomedullin, and only a handful of research labs offer it. These facts notwithstanding, adrenomedullin remains the single best lab test for prognosis in cancer patients.) Other scalar wave benefits include these:

Reduction of free radicals, inflammation, and blood sugar.

Reduction of congenital cartilage tumors.

Increase of Delta brainwave activity, enabling deep relaxation.

Does it matter if we use machines or our minds? The fact is, we can gather and focus scalar energy through our own mental intention. Using a variant of autogenic training, repeat the following in twenty-minute sessions:

As you breathe in, say to yourself, "I breathe ..."
As you breathe out, say "... the power of God."

With each completed breath, give your full belief to the words, "I breathe ... the power of God." Believe and accept that, with each breath, you are calling in and expressing the universal power to heal every cell in your body (or to heal a specific problem).

By this exercise, you'll be doing what spiritual healers like Olga Worrall have done for others and what you have the divine right and native ability to do for yourself: That is, to gather and focus the infinite healing power of scalar energy. And remember: Every time you breathe, you take into yourself the scalar space-equivalent of trillions of helium molecules. Scalar energy surrounds you and is in you, waiting to be focused for healing. With the right intention, you have the power to heal anyone and anything!

In *The Heart of Health: The Principles of Physical Health and Vitality* (Plainview, NY: Natural Healing House, 2003), Stephen Linsteadt and Maria Elena Boekemeyer explain:

> We are all connected to each other and to the energy source that makes up the Universe. We are totally interdependent. Our body, our brain, our consciousness are inextricably joined with other matter in the Universe. Every atom and molecule within us depends on the rest of the Universe. Our brain and other parts of our neural physiology are interconnected by this unseen communication network which coordinates and regulates behavior of certain parts of the body. The body, therefore, can be seen as a dense medium holding the real essence of who we are: Divine energy. We are interconnected outward expressions of this Divine energy.... The manifestation of this energy comes from the empty vacuum, known as the quantum vacuum, which is actually packed full of God's creative energy in a stable state. This all-pervading energy is sometimes referred to as a universal scalar wave, which is a form of electrostatic energy that has the potential to create but is currently without physical manifestation. Potential is only manifested when we provide the frequency information through our thoughts and intentions

of what it is we want to create. This is the concept of mind over matter. (p. 9)

We're aware that skeptics dyed-in-the-wool will have problems with this phenomenon.[23] (This is one instance where the FFT trait of openness might be of benefit.) Though we approach CAM modalities like scalar wave with scientific rigor, we're quite willing to embrace what we've seen with our own eyes, even if we can't yet explain it fully. This "seeing is believing" attitude is the ground of common sense, is it not? So we accept our intuitions and cheerfully declare ourselves pragmatists in energy medicine: What matters most is that *it works*.

Within our holistic model, we've introduced CAM techniques/technologies for mind (autogenic training),

---

23 Linsteadt and Boekemeyer give a more science-based description:

> Scalar waves are produced when two electromagnetic waves of the same frequency are exactly out of phase (opposite to each other) and the amplitudes subtract and cancel or destroy each other. The result is not exactly an annihilation of magnetic fields but a transformation of energy back into a scalar wave. This scalar field has reverted back to a vacuum state of potentiality. Scalar waves can be created by wrapping electrical wires around a figure eight in the shape of a Möbius coil. When an electric current flows through the wires in opposite directions, the opposing electromagnetic fields from the two wires cancel each other and create a scalar wave. The DNA antenna in our cells' energy production centers (mitochondria) assumes the shape of what is called a super-coil. Supercoil DNA look like a series of Möbius coils. These Möbius supercoil DNA are hypothetically able to generate scalar waves. Most cells in the body contain thousands of these Möbius supercoils, which are generating scalar waves throughout the cell and throughout the body. (pp. 9-10)

body (Gamma PEMF), and spirit (scalar wave) combined. As you proceed through the Shealy-Sorin protocols, you'll become further acquainted with these and other modalities of energy medicine; you'll meet other self-assessment tools and other instances where health (in all its aspects) and personality converge. But, throughout, the bottom line remains self-knowledge: *Gnothi se auton,* as the Delphic Oracle advised. Self-knowledge is both a symptom *and* consequence of conscientiousness. That same self-knowledge is both the goal *and* starting point of medical diagnosis. It both precedes *and* results from the various inventories supplied in this chapter. And, as we shall seek to demonstrate, it is strengthened by the health protocols outlined in chapters following.

Wisdom Be Not Proud
(Truth Be Never Cowed)

Truth stood before me
Desiring to see
While pondering,
"Why do you continue ignoring *me*?
Too busy you may say—
Too preoccupied *again* today!
Enamored of programmed current views
Too addicted to the constant news."

Truth stood behind me as I scurried by.
Felt a tug of guilt—
I knew not why.
But then again I knew that *I knew.*
Had I not been in the presence *of what is true?*

Truth sighed and smiled.
"How they do ignore me.
Yet some—a few—
Choose the wisdom path
And with humility
They come to explore me.
Seeking the prudent and far-sighted path
They desire to embrace, esteem ... and adore me."

                                        —**Georgianne Ginder**

CHAPTER THREE

The Shealy-Sorin Protocols: CAM Approaches for Health, Happiness, and Longevity

C. Norman Shealy and Sergey Sorin

In the 14th century, when the word "disease" first appeared in medieval English, it had nothing whatsoever to do with medicine: Referring to the anxious cares of life, it meant "uneasiness" (that is, the *absence* of ease), "disturbance," and "trouble." Only later would it stand for illness as a medical condition. Today, holistic practitioners have sought to restore its original meaning as *dis-ease*—as the lack of physical, emotional, social, spiritual equilibrium in life. A life lived joyfully, healthily, lovingly, peacefully is a life lived "easily." And *dis-ease* is its opposite: a life of anxious cares, disturbances, and troubles. Our holistic approach acknowledges that *dis-ease* leads to disease. Sadly, most Americans live in a near-constant state of *dis-ease*: imbalanced, restless, care-worn, anxious, and unhappy. We'd go so far as to declare *dis-ease* an American lifestyle, one grounded in stress, bad choices, bad habits, and dangerous behaviors—a lifestyle lacking in conscientiousness.

The cure for *dis-ease* is not medical. It can't be cured by alcohol or drugs (prescription or otherwise), though these seem to offer temporary escape. We can't work or worry our way out of it. We can't buy or consume our way out of it. We can't marry or sire our way out of it. A vacation or a change of scenery or of occupation or of spouse might seem to offer respite, *but it will come back*, so long as our lives lack physical, emotional, social, spiritual centeredness, stability, and equilibrium. Individually and collectively, we have a choice to make. We can live in *dis-ease* and allow the stresses of live to spiral downward into physical-mental-emotional-spiritual disease. Or we can choose to live conscientiously. Gentle reader: If you choose the latter, you already know where to start. You'll be mindful of lifestyle choices that optimize health and wellness. You'll eat nutritiously, maintain a healthy weight, avoid smoking, and get plenty of exercise and plenty of sleep.

> Choose feeling happy
> Over feeling crappy.
> Put a voice to your choice—
> And make it snappy!
> —**Georgianne Ginder**

You'll remember that two of the five health essentials that we've been preaching focus on eating habits. If you keep a body mass index of 18 to 24 and eat a minimum of five servings daily of fruits and veggies, you've got a good start at conscientious self-care. Before we go into detail, here's some simple advice: Keep your diet "lean and green" (focusing on lean protein and fruits and veggies) and limit your intake of simple carbohydrates and sugars, including sodas (whether naturally or artificially sweetened). And if you find it hard to eat "lean and green," just remember what's at stake: Proper nutrition can radically reduce incidents of degenerative disease, including heart disease (75%), cancer (78%), respiratory ailments and infection (79%), and diabetes (52%).[1]

Diet, however, is just the starting point. An "informed consumer" (of food, as well as of medical advice) should understand "the science of food": that is, "the processes by which the organism ingests, digests, absorbs, transports, utilizes and excretes food substances." That's a fancy AMA definition for a seemingly simple term, *nutrition.* And food, the AMA reminds us, "consists of proteins, carbohydrates, fats, and other substances (minerals, vitamins and

---

1 See Helen Guthrie, *Introductory Nutrition* (St. Louis, MO: Times Mirror/Mosby College Publishing, 1986). The following paragraphs draw on Guthrie, as well as a series of books by Howard F. Loomis, Jr. These include Loomis's *Enzymes: The Key to Health Volume 1: The Fundamentals* (Madison, WI: 21ˢᵗ Century Nutrition Publishing. 1999), *The Enzyme Advantage: For Health Care Providers and People Who Care About Their Health* (Madison, WI: 21ˢᵗ Century Nutrition Publishing, 2015), and *The Enzyme Advantage: For Women* (Madison, WI: 21ˢᵗ Century Nutrition Publishing, 2016).

enzymes) that are essential for an organism to sustain growth, repair, and to furnish energy for all activity of the organism." The following discussion may seem simple. It's meant to be. Some readers may know some of the following. But don't think of it as "food science for dummies." Unless you're a dietician or physician, we predict that you'll learn a thing or two about the roles nutrition and digestion play in health.

1. Health / Nutrition / Digestion.

Let's start with the macronutrients: carbohydrates, fats, and proteins. Carbohydrates are the body's primary energy supply. Lipids—fats—supply energy, too, but they also provide components of cell membranes and the lipotropic hormones (including the sex hormones). Proteins are essential for energy, cellular growth and repair, and proper functioning of central nervous system components (including such neurotransmitters as dopamine, which affects alertness and motor function, and serotonin, which affects mood and relaxation). Plasma proteins maintain the homeostasis of extracellular fluids in the body. Proteins are also essential in the production of insulin, epinephrine, thyroxine (tied to thyroid function), hemoglobin (tied to blood formation) and antibodies (tied to the immune system).

Generalized symptoms of deficiency in one or more of these macronutrients include stiff and sore joints, headaches, heartburn, indigestion, gas and bloating, constipation, anxiety, depression, and other mood disorders like insomnia and restlessness.

Symptoms of protein deficiency include the following:
Increased secretions in the mouth, nose and eyes.
Swelling in the hands and feet.
Cold hands and feet.
Muscle cramps at night.
Menstrual cramps.
Bleeding gums.
Inability to tolerate exercise.

Carbohydrate deficiency symptoms include these:
Decreased secretions in the mouth nose and eyes.
Water loss and dehydration.
Inability to concentrate.
Muscle cramps during exercise.
Muscle weakness.
Being easily startled.
Fatigue and loss of energy.

Lipid deficiency symptoms include the following:
Dry skin.
Tremors.
Prostaglandin deficiency.
Inability to control blood pressure (high or low).
Difficulty with pregnancy (inducing labor, as well as having spontaneous abortions).

Those are the macronutrients. It's not by eating them simply, but by digesting them that we let them do their work. So, let's talk about the digestive process from the time that the food enters the mouth, until it leaves from the other end.[2]

When food enters the mouth, pre-digestion begins. The term, "pre-digestion," is a misnomer, since it's an important first process in the digestive system. The saliva that fills our mouths is filled with enzymes, including amylase (for carbohydrate digestion), protease (for the metabolism of protein), and lipase (for digestion of fats). When your mother told you, "Slow down, don't wolf your food!" she was giving excellent dietary advice. By chewing slowly and fully, we give these salivary enzymes time to coat the food and start the digestive process. Taking the time to chew also activates chemical receptors in the mouth that trigger our enjoyment of food. (This last point should remind us of the pleasures resting in healthy habits: Eating is a social, spiritual, and emotional activity that affects the whole person. So remember, enjoyment is both a cause and an effect of healthy digestion!)

> **Start with Your pH.** A good starting point in self-diagnosis is your body's acidity level, which you can check via a simple pH strip test of your saliva. Ideally, your pH will be 7.2 to 7.4.

---

2 For an earlier version of this discussion, see Shealy and Sorin, *30 days to Self-Health*.

If you already are eating 80% of your food as veggies and fruits, but your pH is low (that is, too acidic), add one-half to one teaspoon daily of potassium gluconate.

Many decades ago—long before the current fad of "alkaline diets"—the great American medical psychic, Edgar Cayce (1677-1945), declared that "80% of all food eaten should be alkaline-reacting and only 20% acid-reacting" (Shealy, *Energy Medicine* p. 89). Generations of naturopaths have since been weaned on Cayce's work.

After the mouth stage, the swallowed food enters the esophagus where it transitions down towards the upper part of the stomach. When the swallowing goes well we don't normally give it much attention; but when there are esophageal spasms, hiatal hernia, or other dysfunctions, one may experience the sourness and burn of gastroesophageal reflux disease (GERD), whose pains can mimic symptoms of heart attack. (That's why it's called "heartburn," right?)

Before food enters it, the stomach is initially flat. The arrival of the food leads to the stretching of the stomach, which stimulates production of hydrochloric acid (HCl). Under normal circumstances it takes forty-five minutes for stomach acid to form and do its digestive work. As we age, HCl production slows. People over forty need extra time for stomach digestion; people over 65 need an hour or more. (You can see why eating slowly—and chewing fully—can be so important: It gives the salivary enzymes time to get the digestive process under way.)

Here, too, digestion has its psychosocial as well as its physiological components. While the autonomic, sympathetic, and parasympathetic nervous systems all contribute to the stomach phase of digestion, HCl secretion is regulated largely by the parasympathetic system—that is, by the "relaxation phase" of our nervous system cycle. (You can see how Americans' restless "eat-and-run" habits affect mind *and* mood *and* body at once. In the animal kingdom, the lion gorges and then sleeps: For humans, too, an after-dinner nap works wonders for digestion.) HCl secretion has hormonal factors, as well: Gastrin is a peptide hormone involved in HCl production as well as in pepsinogen secretion. Pepsinogen is an inactive form of an enzyme that HCl converts into pepsin—and it's pepsin that begins the process of converting protein into amino acids. (The essential amino acids are phenylalanine; the three branched-chain amino acids valine, leucine, and isoleucine; lysine; threonine; tryptophan; and methionine.)

Contrary to popular belief, too much acid is not the cause of stomach troubles; rather, it's that acid is not adequately produced. Among other stomach ailments, ulcers are marked by a loss of balance between factors that protect the stomach mucosa versus the offending factors that cause mucosal destruction. The mucosal lining is made of water, electrolytes, and glycoproteins. It functions to trap pathogens, coat the walls of the intestine, and aid in forming fecal matter. Being itself resistant to digestive acids, the mucosal lining buffers small amounts of acid and alkaline that keep our gastrointestinal pH in balance.

Thus, the TV commercials hawking stomach acid suppressors couldn't be further from the truth. We need stomach acid! In effect, it "cooks" our food, killing the bacteria that enters the body with the food we've eaten. Inhibiting stomach acid production with antacids interferes with the body's natural defense mechanisms. Antacids aren't "noble firefighters," as portrayed on TV; rather, they're a byproduct of our "sick care" system, which (mis) treats symptoms while ignoring the underlying causes. So much for our misunderstood and much maligned stomach acids ...

From the stomach, food enters the small intestine, the first area of which is the duodenum. There, Brunner's glands secrete mucus as a protection against the acidic juices entering from the upper stomach. And here, too, our lifestyles impact our nervous systems, which impair our digestion: When excess stress activates the sympathetic nervous system—which triggers the "fight or flight" reflex— there's a decrease in mucus production, which can lead to the formation of duodenal ulcers. Instead of fighting acid, we should be reducing stress!

The stomach's acid juices activate bile, an alkaline compound produced in the liver and stored in the gallbladder (which acts like a pouch, holding this vital ingredient for digestion). Normally, the gallbladder will contract as one eats, secreting its bile into the small intestine. The bile serves to emulsify fats, readying them for the digestion. (Think of emulsification as a kind of degreasing mechanism that enables digestive enzyme penetration. Without the proper amount of bile salts, lipids will not be properly digested.)

Given the intense pain of gallstones, gallbladder surgeries are a common emergency room procedure. But cholecystectomy—surgical removal of the gallbladder—rarely solves the underlying dysfunction. Despite the pain of gallbladder contraction when stones are formed, cholecystectomy is the sort of surgery that treats symptoms, not causes. Interestingly, the body will form another pouch to store its bile salts, similar in function to the gallbladder; and if the dysfunction that led to gallstones is not addressed, the symptoms will recur!

It's worth noting that if the stomach does not produce enough acid or if its acid is suppressed (Tums, anyone?), then bile secretion is reduced in turn, leading to poor protein and fat metabolism. In addition, secretin and cholecystokinin are activated by stomach acid in the duodenum. These essential hormones send messages to the pancreas and the biliary portion of the liver that help regulate the amount of the undigested protein, carbohydrates, and fat still present in the chyme (food substrate making its way down the GI tract).

The duodenum also receives pancreatic enzymes via a duct connecting the pancreas to the duodenum. Pancreatic enzymes include protease (which breaks down proteins); amylase (which breaks down starch glycogen into simple sugars like sucrose, lactose for dairy, and maltose for grains); and lipase (which breaks down neutral fats into glycerol, which dissolves further into glucose and fatty acids). Natural/organic plant food sources have their own internal enzymes, which assist the human digestive process. When these natural foods are highly processed and sent off to the supermarket, their enzymes are destroyed. Since most Americans eat processed foods deficient in natural enzymes, we see yet another lifestyle-impact upon digestion: The pancreas is forced to produce even more enzymes, increasing stress that can lead, ultimately, to burn-out.

The second part of the small intestine is the jejunum, where pancreatic enzymes and bile salts do the work of digesting proteins and lipids. Digestion of carbohydrates, however, cannot be completed by pancreatic enzymes alone. The most that they can do is break the long polysaccharide chains of carbs down into disaccharides or "double sugars," in which two monosaccharide molecules (e.g., lactose, maltose and sucrose) are held together by a glycolic bond. Secreting the enzymes lactase, maltase, and sucrase, it's the jejunal microvilli that break these disaccharides down into glucose.

The jejunal microvilli are minute, fingerlike projections from the mucosal cell lining of the intestinal wall; these serve to expand the intestinal lining's total surface area, thereby maximizing cellular absorption of nutrients. When there's any dysfunction of the intestinal lining (or when a diet contains too many carbohydrates), then lactose and maltose can remain undigested, leading to gas and diarrhea. (While sucrose can be absorbed across the gut wall, it cannot be turned into energy and winds up causing stress and constipation.) Among the more serious intestinal dysfunctions is celiac disease. Once again, the Third Party conspires with the American lifestyle to increase stress, indigestion, and malabsorption. Think back to our discussion of GMOs and Roundup, where celiac sprue (among other medical conditions) correlates with glyphosate poisoning. Virtually unheard of a generation ago, as many as one in twenty Americans today suffer from some level of gluten intolerance.

How could a chronic medical condition arise seemingly out of nowhere? Well, it *did* come from somewhere: Chemical poisoning and genetic alteration of our food supply have damaged, and will continue to damage, the digestive systems of many Americans. In celiac disease, the ingestion of wheat gluten causes an autoimmune response, releasing inflammatory chemicals that attack and, over time, destroy the intestinal villi and protective mucosal lining: This leads to malabsorption of nutrients and "leaky gut," among other conditions. Not everyone (thank goodness) is genetically predisposed to celiac sprue and similar autoimmune/digestive dysfunctions. But something in the environment "triggered" their medical conditions: They're like the proverbial "canary in a coal mine," warning us of already-present dangers in our environment and food supply. (Don't eat, drink, or breathe in poison: *That's common sense, right?* But how can we exercise common sense, when poisons literally rain down on us and are encoded genetically into our seed stocks?)

Let's return to a model of healthy digestion. The process of digestion is completed in the small intestine, with the absorption of amino acids, monosaccharides, and fatty acid molecules; crossing the intestinal wall barrier, these enter the blood stream and/or lymphatic circulation, where they'll become the body's energy supply, building blocks for growth and repair, and tools for neurological processes. Indeed, the intestines (both small and large) are the site of production of many essential hormones—including the central nervous system's neurochemicals—all essential for mental function and mood.

And we're not done yet. The large intestine has further roles to play in water absorption and fecal matter formation. These sound like simple tasks, compared to the complex digestive processes of the stomach and small intestine. Still, the large intestine has much to teach us about symbiosis in human biology. We're used to thinking of ourselves as individuals—as separate, independent, living beings. Yet the individual is a complex organization of differentiated interdependent cells, each doing the work to which it's been assigned genetically. Each has its own metabolic processes: The oxygen "we" breathe, the foods "we" eat, the liquids "we" drink are for the sake of cellular respiration. And each cell creates its own waste products needing removal. Can you guess how many cells make up the average adult human? Ten *trillion,* according to the American Society for Microbiology. Though the totals of human vs. nonhuman cells remain conjectural,[3] a ratio of 10:1 bacterial to human cells is commonly accepted. So, the average adult is host to one hundred trillion bacterial cells, *most of which live in the large intestine.*

We have learned to think of the planet as a single, organic, interrelated biosphere. (The philosophy of holism holds for the planet as well as the community and the person.) We are, individually, a permeable biome within a biosphere—a human microcosm within a planetary macrocosm. The bacteria residing in our bowels can be beneficial or detrimental to health, depending on their nature and the microenvironment that hosts them. Under healthy conditions, the bacteria population feeds off of undigested dietary residue and intestinal secretions; in return, the intestinal bacteria produce vitamins and short-chain fatty acids that we human hosts are not able to produce ourselves. It's classic symbiosis, each (ideally) benefitting from the other. Indeed, we're dependent upon our "intestinal flora" (as it's commonly called) for many essential nutrients.

When the bacterial balance is deficient or the intestinal

---

3 Ron Sender, Shai Fuchs, and Ron Milo, "Revised Estimates for the Number of Human and Bacteria Cells in the Body," *PLOS Biology* 14 (2016): e1002533.

microenvironment is inconducive to health, the wrong sorts of bacteria can move in, creating infections and inflammation. You'll remember one of the first pieces of advice given in this chapter: to limit your intake of simple carbohydrates and sugars. It's commonsensical to do so. But we avoid sugars not just to maintain healthy weight: An excess of undigested simple sugars leads to an overgrowth of *candida albicans*—that is, to yeast infection in the gut. We want to maintain a healthy intestinal flora, since the "good bacteria" helps keep the "bad bacteria" out. That's why probiotics and prebiotics are important dietary supplements: By supporting our healthy flora, they help us in "colonization resistance"—that is, they help keep pathogens from establishing themselves in the gut and causing disease.

Since the colon absorbs both vitamin B12 and magnesium, we need to consider the transit time of feces through the large intestine. Individuals with rapid transit times absorb less optimal amounts of these essential minerals, requiring supplementation. With consideration of "transit time," we've reached the final stage of our journey through the GI system: elimination and excretion. The main question to ask: Is it normal (that is, healthy), too fast, or too slow? The generally healthy standard is to have one or two bowel movements a day. Fast elimination—defined as more than twice a day—indicates poor absorption as well as poor utilization of nutrients. Slow excretion—fewer than one bowel movement per day—indicates constipation, whose symptoms include a hardening of stool, straining in passing stools, abdominal pains and cramping, feelings of bloat, and nausea. Like other GI issues, constipation has its psychosocial as well as its physiological causes and consequences. Bad eating habits—lack of dietary fiber from fruits and veggies, for example—can cause constipation. So can lack of exercise. (Those are two of our five health essentials, right?) So can dehydration: Drinking too little liquids (or the wrong kinds) can constipate us. Depression can be both a cause and a consequence. And medications are major culprits in their side effects: opiates, antidepressants, calcium channel blockers (used in some blood pressure medicines), and some antacids can stop us up. This, indeed, is one of the real horrors of opioid addiction: The addict can't poop! The inflammation and degenerative diseases implicated in chronic constipation lead us to one obvious conclusion: Constipation is no mere inconvenience but a potentially serious health issue. It's also a symptom of unhealthy lifestyle and general lack of common sense.

In sum: When we treat ourselves right—taking the five health essentials as our starting point—we'll see real benefits in our digestion and overall GI health. We'll be taking care of our intestinal flora, and our flora will take care of us. And we'll be able to congratulate ourselves for such conscientious self-care. But, when our lifestyle habits—in diet especially—get out of control, our digestion will suffer: We can expect an invasion of "bad bacteria," of yeast and other fungi, and of a horde of viruses, each dumping its toxic waste products into our systems. (In many cases, it's not the "colonization" so much as the toxic metabolites of these biome invaders that make us very, *very* sick.)

Leaky gut syndrome (LGS) is but one of several chronic conditions resulting from imbalances in the gut biome. (Irritable bowel syndrome and Crohn's disease can be added to this list, as can celiac sprue.) In LGS, a weakening of the intestinal mucosal barrier can lead to inflammation and breaks in the protective intestinal wall, allowing toxins and infectious agents to invade the bloodstream and lymphatic system. In battling these invaders, the body has two main defenders, the liver and the immune system. As P. Kubes and C. Jenne write,

> The liver is a key, frontline immune tissue. Ideally positioned to detect pathogens entering the body via the gut, the liver appears designed to detect, capture, and clear bacteria, viruses, and macromolecules. Containing the largest collection of phagocytic cells in the body, this organ is an important barrier between us and the outside world. Importantly, as portal blood also transports a large number of foreign but harmless molecules (e.g., food antigens), the liver's default immune status is anti-inflammatory or immunotolerant; however, under appropriate conditions, the liver is able to mount a rapid and robust immune response. This balance between immunity and tolerance is essential to liver function. (p. 247)[4]

---

4 P. Kubes and C. Jenne, "Immune Responses in the Liver," *Annual Review of Immunology* 26 (2018): 247-77. They continue: "Excessive inflammation in the absence of infection leads to sterile liver injury, tissue damage, and remodeling; insufficient immunity allows for chronic infection and cancer. Dynamic interactions between the numerous populations of immune cells in the liver are

The liver has a remarkable capacity for self-regeneration. When poor lifestyle choices—including chronic alcoholism and abusive drug use (prescription or otherwise)—push this miraculous organ beyond its limits, then liver function and structure will be compromised and eventually decompensate and fail.

The immune system consists of the thymus and bone marrow (these being the primary lymphoid organs), as well as the spleen, tonsils, lymph vessels, lymph nodes, adenoids, and skin (these being the secondary lymphatic tissues). If you think of the body as a defensive fortification, these organs and tissues would serve as its earthworks and ramparts, protecting against threats external as well as internal. A healthy immune system does a remarkable job in detecting, capturing, and removing toxins. Like the liver, however, it too can be overrun and brought to exhaustion. Put simply, our immune systems wage a constant daily battle against environmental biotoxins and chemicals in the air, food, and water. It doesn't help that we let in these toxic invaders of our own accord. Through a lack of conscientiousness, we eat foods contaminated with growth hormones and pesticides; we drink polluted, fluoridated water; we breathe in fumes from nearby factories and their chemical waste dumps; we live under the EMF pollution of power lines and transformers. Even when we think we're being relatively healthy and conscientious, toxins creep in. That innocent box of cereal or protein bar may contain

key to maintaining this balance and overall tissue health" (p. 247).

a GMO-contaminated food source: Unwary of dangers hidden inside, we give it entry like a Trojan Horse.

When the immune system begins to malfunction or fail, there is significant potential for developing allergies, chemical sensitivities, and frequent infections as well as autoimmune diseases. We've already mentioned celiac sprue: Triggered by wheat gluten, the celiac suffer's immune system turns against the body's own cells and organs. (In the celiac's case, it's the intestinal mucosa and villi that are attacked and destroyed.) An inflammatory response is a common means of immune-system defense. In rheumatoid arthritis—yet another chronic inflammatory condition—the body attacks its own synovium (that is, the tissue-membranes protecting one's joints). Chronic inflammation causes the synovium to thicken, which leads in time to the destruction of cartilage and bone. The AMA and medical community generally have no explanation: They can give the symptoms but not the cause. Well, *we know* that it's environmental, that it's triggered by something in what we eat, drink, or breathe in. And if we were to take bets, we'd place our money on pesticides.[5]

Autoimmune dysfunction can set off a vicious cycle of susceptibility to infections, which leads to an overreliance on antibiotics and other drugs and pharmaceuticals, which can wipe out "good bacteria" in the gut, which can lead to further infectious processes and inflammatory conditions (like IBS and Crohn's disease), and so on ...

---

5 See Armando Meyer et al., "Pesticide Exposure and Risk of Rheumatoid Arthritis among Licensed Male Pesticide Applicators in the Agricultural Health Study," *Environmental Health Perspectives*, 14 July 2017 (https://www.ncbi.nlm.nih.gov/pmc/articles/PMC5744649/), accessed 14 February 2020.

An "Inflammation Nation": Healing and Hate

Can one be healed whilst harboring hate?
Must a healer not evaluate—?
Treading the path of reconciliation,
The balm dissolving inflammation.

Making a living—
Producing *more*
Weapons, pollutants, toxins
By the score.

Such production takes its toll
On spirit, body, mind, and soul.
Can one be healed when one neglects
The very truth that one rejects?

To fear what all will come to be,
Denying *life* eternally,
Yet still that small voice speaks anew
Reminding all of what is true.

                    —Georgianne Ginder (March 19, 2015)

Some Further Food Advice.

You already know to avoid wheat, sugar, and fast food restaurants. In your food choices, you want to keep the pH ratio of 80% alkaline foods to 20% acidic foods. Now, most fruits (excepting citrus) and veggies are alkaline, while most protein and carbohydrates are acidic. That gives you a starting point: Try to keep your diet 80% fruits and veggies and 20% protein and carbs. You've heard of the classic "square meal," consisting of a protein, a starch (typically potato), and one vegetable. That doesn't cut it for the 21st century! In any meal, try not to mix proteins and carbs (e.g., steak and potatoes). Instead, combine protein with fruit/veggies. If you want to have a carbohydrate, try a baked sweet potato combined with fruits/veggies. Limiting portion size can be helpful: Portions in restaurants (and even homecooked meals) tend to be piled on. Put less on your plate! You can go back for seconds if you choose. Intermittent fasting or changing your scheduled mealtimes can give your GI tract a much-needed break and chance to recover. For example, eat two meals per day, with breakfast at 6am and dinner at 6pm and no food intake (no snacking!) in between these twelve-hour intervals. (Breakfast can be thought of as "breaking one's overnight fasting.") And the best-ever breakfast is a morning slush with 24 to 36 grams of whey protein, 2 tablespoons of beef gelatin, a heaping teaspoon of Berry Fusion, a packet of Kyani Sunrise and 2 tablespoons of tart cherry juice concentrate, giving you whopping 14,500 ORACS (antioxidants) to start your health day. Eating no later than two hours before bedtime is another helpful way to allow better digestion and prevent reflux. If you need further guidance, there are commercial diet plans—the Atkins Diet, South Beach Diet, and Weight Watchers among others—that balance healthy proteins with vegetables (plus or minus fruits). There are many ways to achieve healthy nutrition!

In caring for your health, you can always start with conventional medicine. In acute illnesses, conventional medicine may save your life. But, if the treatment suggested does not work or you evaluate the risks and are not willing to take them, then CAM approaches (call them what you will: complementary, alternative, holistic, integrative) offer a strong, tried-and-true safety net. The Shealy-Sorin Wellness Institute continues the work of Dr. Shealy's original holistic clinic which, over the years, has helped over 32,000 patients for whom mainstream medicine failed. The following paragraphs give a sense of the size and efficacy of the modern "holistic medicine cabinet." Specific Conditions (ADHD, alcoholism, allergies, Alzheimer's, arthritis, autoimmune diseases, etc.) are listed, along with their holistic/homeopathic/bioenergetic remedies.

2. Vitamins / Minerals / Supplements.

When the minimal daily requirements for vitamins and minerals was set over seventy years ago, the world was far less polluted. Even in the late 1970s, Emanuel Cheraskin had demonstrated that the optimal intake of vitamin C was 1000 mg instead of the RDA of 60 mg. Vitamins A, C and E and other antioxidants are essential for dopamine, serotonin, and most brain and body functions. (Interestingly, black pepper is useful for maintaining anandamide, the "bliss" hormone.)

Everyone needs the basic vitamins: B1, B2, B3, B6, folic acid, B12, vitamin A (especially astaxanthin), vitamin C, vitamin D3, vitamin E as tocotrienols, vitamin K2, Omega 3 essential fatty acids, boron, potassium, magnesium, and selenium. Throughout this book, we've been preaching "the five health essentials," one of which is a healthy diet that includes at least five servings of fruits and vegetables per day. Let's admit that we don't always make it to five; besides, the nutritional value of most supermarket produce has severely eroded over recent decades. To compensate, you should consider supplementing with some powdered "super greens." There are many on the market, but we particularly like Zija Core Moringa Super Mix. Taken daily, each packet contains the equivalent antioxidants of 5 servings of veggies. Some additional recommendations follow. But even "super greens" aren't enough. The next list— including two different multivitamins, vitamin D3, magnesium lotion, and copper/zinc—isn't all that long, but it provides a foundation for health in the 21ˢᵗ century.

> **Moringa Oleifera:** The miracle tree. This plant has more generalized health benefits than all other foods combined! Indeed, it has been said that this supplement alone could replace a majority of the usual supplements taken! Moorings has the highest ORAC (antioxidant) content in the world,

1575 ORACS in one gram. It is twice as high as the runner-up Acai berries.

It has higher protein than milk; higher potassium than bananas, higher calcium than milk; higher magnesium than eggs; 50 times the B3 of peanuts; 50 time the B2 of bananas; 7 times the C of oranges; 4 times the vitamin A of carrots. However, there is one and only one product that has it all: Zija Core Moringa Supermix. This contains leaves, seed and fruit and is the single greatest contributor to great energy, This Super Mix of the number one superfood has 13 grams of powder, providing a whopping 6400 ORACS (antioxidants) equal to six servings of ordinary fruits and vegetables, and only 40 calories! If everyone added just this every day, they would have all the essential fruits and vegetable needed! Indeed, this is our unequivocal recommendation for all people.

Here are some of Moringa's outstanding health/medical benefits:

Antidepressant
Anticancer
Anti-inflammatory
Cures colitis, including ulcerative, Irritable bowel and collagenous

Detoxifies
Eliminates constipation
Improves digestion
Improves wound healing
Improves peptic ulcers
Improves skin health
Improves mental clarity and alertness
improves vision
Increases energy and endurance
Lowers cholesterol
Lowers blood sugar
Reduces blood pressure
Strengthens immune system
Reduces pain of all kinds

The Shealy-Sorin "basic essentials" follow, all of which are available from the Wellness Institute (see Appendix for contact information).

Shealy Essentials: First, *everyone* needs a good basic multivitamin (MVI) even more so today, given the increasing oxidation stresses of world pollution. There are many brands besides our own proprietary blend; whatever you choose, make sure that it has at least 25 to 50 mg of the B vitamins (not including B12). B Complex is essential for energy, metabolism, and proper absorption of other vitamins/supplements. If you are not taking a good MVI or if you are not sure about the one you are taking, check the label. If it doesn't have B complex of 25 to 50 mg, then take two capsules daily of Dr. Shealy's Eco-Green Iron-Free Essentials Multivitamin.

Shealy Youth Formula: In addition to Shealy Essentials (or a good MVI with B complex), this is the next most important supplement for everyone. Its patented formula contains 2 gm of vitamin C, essential for immune system and complementary to the B complex in Shealy Essentials. Dr. Shealy's Youth Formula also contains Molybdenum and MSM in a proprietary, patented combination that raises DHEA (Dehydroepiandrosterone), the essential health hormone for youthful longevity. Dose for adults is 4 capsules per day.

Vitamin D3: Vitamin D3 is essential for bone health, as well as for a proper functioning immune system. It is actually a hormone in itself, important in regulatory functions. Many physicians recognize the need for vitamin D but prescribe D2, which is not nearly as effective as vitamin D3. Furthermore, the right dose for adults is 50,000 units per week if weight is at or greater than 139 pounds; if less than 139 pounds, then take 50,000 units every 10 days or 3 times per month. Vitamin D3 can also be used in case of upper respiratory infection by taking 3 capsules of 50,000 units (150,000 units daily for 3 days), then returning to doses weekly or every 10 days.

Astaxanthin: This form of vitamin A is one of the basic/essential supplements and is especially good for skin, eyes, and immune system support. Depending on your immune system (which plays important role in protection as well as internal detoxification and regulation) the dose is 10 to 30 mg daily.

Magnesium Lotion or Spray: The entire human population is now largely deficient in one of the most essential minerals: Magnesium, which is depleted in the soil, gets depleted in the body by physical/emotional stress, and is poorly absorbed orally. Magnesium plays a role in over 350 metabolic processes of body and brain function. It helps with aches and pains (musculoskeletal); it promotes bone health, cellular health, and mental/emotional health; and it ameliorates chronic illness. Testing for Magnesium with blood work is frequently not accurate, as it is an intracellular element and will show normal on blood chemistry until severe depletion. Many people take Magnesium by mouth, but the best way is transdermal, via magnesium lotion or spray. Applying magnesium directly on an area of pain or tenderness helps relieve pain and tension; by this means, it gets absorbed and used by the body without having to pass through the liver. Absorbed transdermally, magnesium helps produce DHEA, the essential anti-stress "youth" hormone.

We're confident in our clinic's proprietary formula, Dr. Shealy's Biogenics Magnesium Lotion. Adult dose is either 4 tsp of lotion (2 in the morning and 2 at night is best), or 20 sprays. When applying, avoid contact with eyes or other sensitive areas, as magnesium can cause temporary burning sensation on sensitive skin or in eyes.

Copper intake is as essential for health as zinc and is strongly associated with the number one measurement of potential longevity, telomere length.[6]

For Correcting for Deficiencies: DHEA, taurine, methylation.

DHEA support: DHEA (Dehydroepiandrosterone) is an essential hormone produced in the adrenals in response to stress. Cortisol is the primary stress hormone that is released in acute stress reaction; DHEA functions to normalize the Cortisol and body balance after the stress is removed. In chronic stress, and in virtually every physical/emotional malady, DHEA is depleted, leaving the unopposed cortisol (and other stress hormones) to create havoc in the body—including chronic sympathetic "fight or flight" predominance over the parasympathetic "relaxation response."

Some people take oral DHEA supplements, but there is potential concern when taking an exogenous hormone. One exception is those who use prednisone (or other exogenous steroids, as prescribed by their physician), in which case oral DHEA may be helpful. Otherwise, Dr. Shealy and the Shealy-Sorin Wellness Institute have come up with a patented approach to increase DHEA production naturally. There are four means to do so:

> Shealy Youth Formula (see above in basics/ essentials) raises DHEA by 60%.

---

6 See Z. Lin, H. Gao, B. Wang, and Y. Wang, "Dietary Copper Intake and Its Association with Telomere Length: A Population-Based Study," *Frontiers in Endocrinology* 30.9 (2018): 404.

Magnesium Lotion or Spray (see basics/essentials) raises DHEA by 60%.

Eugesterone Cream/Lotion provides progesterone, which can be converted to other essential sex hormones as well as DHEA increase by 60%.

Shealy Fire Bliss essential oil applied to specific acupuncture meridian points helps normalize hormonal function from gonads to adrenals to thyroid to pituitary-thalamic axis while reducing anxiety, depression, and autoimmune disorders.

Taurine Deficiency: Taurine deficiency is common in depression, epilepsy, obesity, macular degeneration, hypercholesterolemia, diabetes, hypertension, congestive heart failure, and most chronic diseases. Its functions are many: It helps regulate cholesterol, protect the kidneys, and moderate the critical movement of sodium, potassium, and magnesium into and out of cells; it contributes to normal brain rhythm, controlling seizures; it balances white blood cell production of free radicals to fight infection; and it enables peak athletic performance.

Taurine is a "conditionally essential" amino acid, as some people cannot manufacture it from methionine and cysteine. Importantly, it can only be found in animal products: *There is no naturally occurring taurine in any plant!* Vegans and the two-thirds of overweight people—and most men—need more taurine, which is also essential for testicular function.

Taurine also works in normalizing the electrical charge across cell membranes. This is especially important in anxiety/depression as well as in labile hypertension, where the normal charge of -70 mV is compromised and may be as low as -20 mV. Taurine works synergistically with magnesium to normalize the electrical charge on nerve cells. Extra taurine is essential in treating epilepsy and hypertension.

Methylation defects are tied to a wide variety of conditions: Addiction, ADHD, allergies, Alzheimer's, anxiety, atherosclerosis, autism, autoimmune diseases, bipolar depression, cancer, chronic viral infections, dementia, diabetes, fibromyalgia, Hashimoto's hypothyroidism, Lyme disease, neuropathy, pulmonary embolism, schizophrenia. Individuals with methylation defects may also have trouble making taurine and run a high homocysteine (above 7.5), with all the consequences thereof. Methylation defects may be helped by taking methyl folate and methylcarbylamine.

Lithium Orotate: Lithium is one of the body's essential components in making Serotonin, which is a neurohormone responsible for mood, as well as for mental functioning during waking hours. Disorders of serotonin lead to anxiety, depression, significant stress, and a host of other mood and mental health disorders. In these conditions, adding lithium helps to stabilize function brain and normalize Serotonin production. Dosage varies from 10 up to 40 mg per day.

Note: Many people have heard of lithium carbonate, a pharmaceutical drug that is based on lithium but is given at much higher doses (900 to 1200 mg per day). The chemical composition and other components of lithium carbonate make it a potentially dangerous drug with significant side effects, whereas lithium orotate in a natural formulation at homeopathic doses carries virtually no side effects and does as good and even better job.

Tryptophan: This amino acid is a chemical precursor in making serotonin, the bright-eyed happy wake-up neurochemical essential for mood, daytime activity, and brain function. As a supplement, it can be instrumental in treatment of mood disorders, especially anxiety and depression.

Dosage ranges from 2 grams to 6 grams per day for severe symptoms. And it should be taken with Shealy Essentials and Lithium orotate.

For Cardiovascular and Metabolic Support: Some minerals and supplements.

Lecithin Granules: Lecithin is a lipid that makes up components of the brain and central nervous system. As a brain support, it aids in mental clarity and in the prevention and treatment of mild to moderate memory problems, including dementia. It also helps to support and normalize cholesterol and the metabolic pathways; hence, it is one of the key regimens for cholesterol or triglyceride dysfunction.

Chromium and Vanadium are trace elements essential for sugar and metabolic support. They are helpful in addressing hyperglycemia, diabetes, and pre-diabetes.

Gymnema Sylvestra is a Chinese herb that lowers blood sugar and aids in diabetes, pre-diabetes, and metabolic syndrome. To fight or suppress sugar or sweet cravings, capsules can be opened and a few grains placed on the tongue. Usual dose is 1 capsule (300 to 400 mg) with each meal, or up to 3 times a day.

Berberine a safe herb that helps lower blood sugar. Dosage ranges from 500 to 1000 mg twice daily.

Gugulipid is a supplement helpful with metabolism, cholesterol, and blood sugar/diabetes.

Typical dose is 400 mg 3 times a day.

For Immune System Support: Vitamins and supplements.

In the Shealy-Sorin Wellness Institute, clients regularly receive intravenous vitamin C (Myer's Cocktails): While the ingredients vary with each person's needs, the typical cocktail contains up to 100 gm of vitamin C plus magnesium, B complex, and B12. This is an essential rejuvenating cocktail for better energy, as well as our primary go-to treatment for an underactive immune system, which can present as poor healing, frequent infections, autoimmune disease, and even cancer (which on one level is a failure of the immune system to deal with abnormal cell growth in the body). The following additional supplements are useful, as well.

Vitamin K2 is an essential companion to vitamin D3. It is present at 100 micrograms in Shealy Essentials, but can be taken in doses of 15 mg for stronger immune support. Because it serves as antidote to Coumadin, people should consult their physician and be careful taking K2 when on blood thinners.

Colostrum: This powder brings the benefit of mother's milk, which supports gastrointestinal immune function. GI track is the primary essential immune organ and proper balance can help normalize many body functions. Usual dose: 1 tsp daily 1 or 2 times per day.

Autoimmune-X: This combination of over 100 compounds supports healthy gastrointestinal function and addresses leaky gut syndrome; taken over 3-6 months, it helps normalize immune function by correcting for too low or too active autoimmune responses. It also improves intercellular communication, and aids in the functioning of virtually all twelve organ systems. (For dosage directions, contact company.)

For Detoxification: Castor oil.

Castor oil is one of the great Edgar Cayce's favorite remedies. It serves a number of functions, including detoxification, immune support, improved healing, and detoxification. Castor oil can be applied topically in a number of ways.

Castor oil suit: Apply castor oil generously over the trunk and lower body and wear an old sweat suit (which can't be used again other than for use with castor oil). Start before bedtime and the castor oil will be absorbed by the time you wake up.

Castor oil sauna: If you have a regular or infra-red sauna, apply castor oil to the body and stay in the sauna for 15-20 minutes. Make sure to wash the body fully afterward.

Castor oil bath: You can put castor oil into a warm bath and absorb castor oil in this way, but be very careful getting out of the tub, as it will be slippery. You'll also have to wash the bathtub afterward (which makes this a more difficult application).

Castor oil eye drops: With any injury or even cataracts of the eyes, use pharmaceutical-grade castor oil (USP), with 1-2 drops once or more per day. This accelerates healing, reverses cataracts, and helps with any pain from superficial injury.

Testing after Age Forty: Controlling cholesterol, A-1c, and cardiac calcium.

If you have excellent health habits and no symptoms, it would be wise by age forty to have a comprehensive metabolic and lipid profile, Hemoglobin A-1c, High sensitivity C Reactive protein, and a calcium score (the simplest, safest test for coronary artery disease) or a CT of the heart. If any of the test results are abnormal, proceed with the following alternatives. If cholesterol is above 200, HDL below 50, or triglycerides over 100, take 2 heaping tablespoons of lecithin granules twice daily and trimethyl glycine 2000 mg three times daily; recheck in four to eight weeks. Remember: If a physician recommends a statin drug, fire him or her! *Never* take a statin drug!

Another problem routinely missed in conventional medicine is prediabetes. It can come upon you up to ten years before the onset of full-blown diabetes, causing neuropathy—numbness and pain in the legs and feet. We recommend getting a Hemoglobin A-1c test as a baseline not later than age 50 and every five years after that. If your HGB A-1c is between 5.6 and 6.4, then you have prediabetes. This needs to be brought under control with stress management, gymnema sylvestra, berberine, fenugreek, and reducing body fat to a healthy BMI of 18 to 24. (Of course, all five of the "basic health essentials" play their part.) Do not be pushed into Metformin or other drugs!

If your cardiac calcium score is above 100, it's time to start a holistic approach to longevity. If you are in the 40ᵗʰ percentile or higher for your age group, then you might consider chelation (described below). And, given your age group, there's a pretty good chance that your dental work included silver-mercury amalgam fillings. If any remain in your teeth, find a competent dentist to remove them.

For Men after Age 50: Recommended supplements.
Adam's Prostate Care, daily.
Zinc chelate, 20 mg daily.
Copper chelate, 4 mg.

Saw Palmetto, 160 mg double strength extract, three times daily.
Boron, 12 mg daily.

Treating ADHD: This disorder is grossly over-diagnosed, and Ritalin should virtually *never* be used! There is never an excuse for Prozac or other mood-altering drugs with this condition. Here are our recommendations:
Vitamin D3 50,000 units once a month in adults 140 pounds or heavier.
Vitamin K2 15 mg daily, and up to 45 mg in serious immune problems.
Shealy Air Bliss on the Ring of Air twice daily.
If this does not work rapidly, add Earth Bliss twice daily.
Lithium orotate 5 to 20 mg daily.
Taurine 1000 to 3000 mg daily.
Dr. Shealy's Biogenics Magnesium Lotion, two teaspoons on skin twice daily (or Magnesium Lotion Spray, 10 sprays twice daily).
Photostimulation with the Shealy RelaxMate II an hour daily.
Biogenics CD: Start with Basic Schultz daily.
Avoid sugar, sodas, and aspartame (artificial sweeteners).

Treating Alcoholism/Addiction: Start with "basic/essentials" (see above) and add the following.

Shealy Earth Bliss on Earth points, plus stimulation
of the addiction points bilaterally, up to twice
daily.
Lithium orotate 45 mg daily
Shealy-Sorin Chakra Sweep Gamma PEMF two hours
daily trans-cranially. This is the only treatment
proven   to stop addiction cravings!
Biogenics program as outlined in 90 Days to Self-
Health.
Past-life therapy.

For Alcoholism/Addiction due to dopamine deficiency:
Dopamine deficiency can cause apathy, fatigue, depression,
severe addictions, ADHD, obesity, and Parkinson's Disease.
*Interestingly, one of the causes of dopamine deficiency
is a high sugar intake!* The amino acid l-phenylalanine
is the precursor for making dopamine. Dopamine-rich
foods alone generally do not have the amino acid levels
necessary to boost levels for someone experiencing major
depressive disorder. Tyrosine supplementation may help.
A healthy sleep schedule of 7 or 8 hours of sleep nightly
assists in the production of dopamine and other positive
neurotransmitters, such as serotonin. Regular exercise,
30 minutes at least 5 days a week, is another essential
for optimal mood. (Beside for being more enjoyable, 30
minutes of exercise is more calming and infinitely safer
than Valium." Start with the "basic/essentials" and add the
following:

Decrease sugar intake.

Tyrosine 1000 mg once or twice daily.

Tri-chromium two capsules daily.

Magnesium lotion 2 teaspoons twice daily.

Black pepper one-half teaspoon daily.

Shealy Earth Bliss on Earth points, plus stimulation of the addiction points bilaterally, up to twice daily.

Lithium orotate 45 mg daily.

Shealy-Sorin Chakra Sweep PEMF two hours daily trans-cranially.

Biogenics program as outlined in 90 Days to Self-Health.

Past-life therapy.

Treating Allergies: Most allergies are at least aggravated by food allergies. Start by avoiding wheat, milk products, eggs, citrus, corn and peanuts, the most common food problems. Add:

Vitamin D3 50,000 units once a week in adults.

Vitamin K2 15mg daily.

Astaxanthin 20 mg daily.

Shealy's Youth Formula 4 daily.

Kyani Sunset 3 tablets daily.

Co-Q10 180 mg daily.

Beta 1,3 glucans 500 mg daily.

Chia seeds, s to 3 tablespoons daily.

Treating Alzheimer's Disease: In ameliorating its symptoms, we recommend the following.

Lecithin Granules, two heaping tablespoons twice daily.

Stimulation of Ring of Fire daily, plus alternate with Ring of Air, Earth, Crystal.

Dr. Shealy's Essentials 2 daily.

Methyl cobalamin at least 1000 mcg, sublingual daily.

Methyl folate 1000 mcg daily.

Vitamin D3 50,000 units once a week.

Vitamin K2 15 to 45 mg daily.

CoQ10 400 mg daily.

Lithium orotate at least 15 mg daily.

Bacopa monnieri 500 mg, 3 daily.

Ashwagandha 500 mg, 3 daily.

Omega-3 fatty acids 3 grams daily.

Cognitol (Om-Chi Herbs) 2 daily.

Mem-For (Om-Chi) 3 daily.

If not eating 10 servings daily of fruits and veggies, take Berry Fusion concentrate powder, 1 heaping teaspoon daily.

Physical exercise, 1 hour daily.

Sapphire-Enhanced AdrenoScalar 8 hours every night.

Shealy-Sorin Gamma PEMF at least 2 hours daily.

Treating Anxiety/Panic Disorder: Treat with "Basics" and add the following.

Shealy Air Bliss on Ring of Air twice daily.

Double the amount of Biogenics Magnesium Lotion.

Read and Practice *90 Days to Self-Health.*

Lithium orotate 15 to 40 mg daily.

If not much improved in 4 weeks, add Liss stimulator transcranially for one hour each morning and the RelaxMate II an hour at bedtime.

Shealy-Sorin Gamma PEMF 2 hours transcranially daily.

Consider 10 shots of magnesium, 75 to 100 grams in Myers cocktail IV, if not better in one month.

Treating Arthritis: A majority of arthritis problems are "osteoarthritis." This implies wear and tear and is sometimes the result of trauma. As a metabolic problem it is extremely variable and to some extent genetically influenced. It may affect just the fingers, or spine, hips, knees, etc. In most instances, it reflects an imbalance between calcium and magnesium, poor pH balance, excess free radicals, and possibly inadequate water intake over many years. Try at least two quarts of non-chlorinated, non-fluoridated water daily. Then add:

Joint Support, one heaping tablespoon and 3 capsules daily.

Zyflammend Whole Body, 2 daily.

Boron 12 to 15 mg daily.

Boswellia 500 mg three times daily.

Curcumin with black pepper, 500 mg three times daily.

Vitamin D3 50,000 units once a week.

Vitamin K2 15 to 45 mg daily.

If you must use an anti-inflammatory drug, try aspirin first. Remember, unless you have allergies, L-glutamine may help greatly with avoiding gastrointestinal complications.

Keep salivary pH at 7.4. Use K-Bicarb up to 1000 mg daily.

Shealy-Sorin chakra sweep PEMF locally for 1 to 2 hours daily.

Treating Asthma: Treat with "Basics" plus Anxiety Disorder plus DHEA restoration. Then add the following:

Magnesium replacement is essential: We recommend Dr. Shealy's Biogenics Magnesium Lotion 2 tsp twice daily.

Vitamin D 50,000 units once a week.

Vitamin K2 15 mg daily.

Consider food allergies as a contributor: Avoid wheat, corn, milk products, eggs, peanuts, and citrus for a month.

Stimulate Ring of Air daily with Shealy Air Bliss and Ring of Crystal with Crystal Bliss.

Treating Autoimmune Diseases: Lupus, rheumatoid arthritis, scleroderma, ulcerative colitis.

Treat with "Basics" as well as immune-enhancing approaches. The Seutermann homeopathic approach (see below) has also been particularly helpful in scleroderma and rheumatoid arthritis.

Especially use D 3, 50,000 units once a week and K 2, 15 to 45 mg daily.

Avoid Wheat gluten as if it were poison!

Using Shealy Bliss oils, stimulation of the Sacred Rings is especially recommended, alternating days with Fire, Earth and Crystal.

Practice the techniques in *90 Days to Self-Health.*

Treating Brain Cancer: To build up the body's resources in fighting the cancer, we recommend the following.

20 IVs of 100 grams of vitamin C in a Myers cocktail, 3 days a week for 7 weeks.

Vitamin D3 50,000 units once a week.

Vitamin K2 45 mg daily.

Work with a spiritual healer.

Treating Heavy Metal Toxicity: To remove heavy metals from the body, we recommend IV chelations for their speed and efficacy. There's also Chelex, an oral form of chelation that some therapists swear by, though the process is slow-going: dosage is 4 capsules daily for one year.

We've mentioned the toxicity of silver-mercury amalgam fillings. These pose a long-term hazard, in that mercury can poison many organ systems in the body. If you have amalgams and concerned about the dangers, you should see a biological dentist who is proficient and expert in safely removing those. (In Springfield, Mo. area there are two dentists whom we recommend Call the Wellness Institute for a referral. And *do not* use a dentist who is hell-bent on fluoride.)

Don't Smoke!

This is by far the simplest, most compelling of all recommendations made in this book: *Stop!* Just stop smoking! Smoking is implicated in at least 50% of all deaths among smokers (and, given the poisons in second-hand smoke, it kills non-smokers as well).

Tobacco contains nicotine, a highly addictive substance harder to quit than narcotics, and at least seventy carcinogenic chemicals. Smoking increases heart disease of all kinds—heart attack, angina pectoris, atrial fibrillation, congestive heart failure—plus allergies, anxiety, asthma, cancer (of bladder, cervix, colon, esophagus, kidney, larynx, lung, mouth, nose, pancreas, sinuses, stomach, or throat). It contributes to depression, erectile dysfunction, increased risk of diabetes, intermittent claudication, emphysema, hypertension, and infertility. If this list sounds bad, we're still not done: Smoking causes increases in all infections, fatigue, loss of taste and smell, low birthweight and miscarriage as well as cleft lip in babies, macular degeneration, stroke, tooth and gum disease (including loss of teeth), thrombi (blood clots and emboli), poor wound healing, skin wrinkling, and premature aging.

By the way, vaping is at least as harmful as smoking! And although medical marijuana is rapidly becoming common, I still think casual marijuana use produces more potheads than geniuses. So: Just say *no*.

Do Exercise!

This next recommendation is simple, too: *Just do it!* Sitting all day is as stressful as smoking a pack of cigarettes daily. If nothing else, stand and walk about two minutes every hour. Or, find something physical that you are willing to do at least thirty minutes five days a week.

Physical Exercise is:

The single best and safest treatment for mild to major depression, even in those resistant to drug therapy!

The single best and safest treatment for anxiety.

It reduces stress, hostility and anger.

It improves cognitive thinking at all ages.

It reduces fibromyalgia symptoms more than any known drug.

It reduces all age mortality, especially from heart disease.

It improves immune function.

It helps prevent Alzheimer's.

It helps maintain healthy weight.

It reduces risk of diabetes.

Our favorite exercise assists are the following:

Health Rider, a bicycle with moving-up-and-down seat and handlebars. You can put 50 pounds or more on the bar under the seat to exercise every muscle below your head.

Confidence Fitness Slim Full Body Vibration Platform Fitness Machine: This vibration trainer increases muscle strength, improves circulation, improves general fitness, increases bone density, prevents and treats osteoporosis, decreases cellulite. If you suffer from joint problems, have a heart condition, or use a pacemaker, we recommend seeking medical advice before using a vibration machine.

You don't need elaborate equipment, however. Dr. Shealy's YouTube video, "Bounce for Health!" is a quick, easy, and cost-free approach to exercise.[7]

Seutermann Homeopathy for rheumatoid arthritis, scleroderma, and other autoimmune disorders.

For rheumatoid arthritis and scleroderma, we strongly recommend the Seutermann Homeopathy approach, which has been researched and supplied by Heel Worldwide of Baden, Germany. (Dr. Shealy spent time in Germany studying with its inventor and recommends the protocol for all autoimmune disorders, including Crohn's disease, lupus, psoriasis, and multiple sclerosis.) Note: To use these preparations, you will need to obtain them through an M.D., D.O., nurse practitioner, or naturopath. Components

---

7   See YouTube video, "Bounce for Health!" (https://www.youtube.com/watch?v=HOz-1GdRCs4), accessed 28 March 2020.

are available from HEEL Inc., exclusive distributor of Heel products in the United States.[8]

The Seutermann approach uses twice weekly:

A Quinone

A Krebs cycle component

A nosode

A detox

A standard homeopath remedy

A disease or organ specific

These are usually given subcutaneously but can be taken orally. A detailed schedule (with ingredients) follows.

1st Week

Glyoxal only

2nd Week

Lymphomyosot

Insektized injeel

Rhodendron

Rheum

Glyoxal

Kreb

Echinacen

Procainum

Ranunculus

---

8   For ordering and contact information, see Appendix below.

Thalamus
Ubichinon—quinone
Kreb

3rd Week
Causticum
Lithium cabonicum injeel
Spascupreel
Placenta
Anthrachinon injeel—quinone
Kreb
China homo.
Zeel
Traumeel
Plumbum metallicum
Methylenblau injeel—quinone
Kreb

4th Week
Cactus
Platinum metallicum injeel
Viscum comp forte
Calcarea fluoride
Tonico napthochinon injeel—quinone
Kreb
Aconitum homo
Valeriana injeel forte
Zeel
Thuja injeel

Glyxal—quinone
Kreb

5th Week
Pulsatilla
Vinum badenase injeel
Thyroidea comp
Traumeel
Chimudron injeel—quinone
Kreb
Strophanthus comp
Selenium homo
Zeel
Aurum
Methylgyoxal injeel-quinone
Kreb

6th Week
Tabacum injeel
Traumeel
Spascupreel
Rheum
Para benzochinon—quinone
Kreb
Sabal
Lymphomysot
Zeel
Traumeel
Hydrochinon injeel ---quinone
Kreb

The above protocol may be repeated indefinitely.[9] We also recommend the Seutermann protocol for general immune strengthening. The following twelve-week program alternates between Monday and Thursday treatments.

1st Week	Monday	Thursday
	Glycol	Methylglyoxal
		Anthrachinon
		Glandular Suprarenaiis
		Tuberculinum
		Alcohol, Inm.
		Argentum Niticum

2nd Week	Monday	Thursday
	Citric Acid	Cisacontic Acid
	Chinhudron	Hydrochinon
	Placenta Comp.	Cerebrum Comp.
	Arsenicum	Lymphomyosot
	Gripheel	Herpes Zoster Nosode
	Cactus Comp.	Cimicifuga Homo.

3rd Week	Monday	Thursday
	Isocitrate	Oxalosuccinic Acid
	Napthochinon	Parabenzochinon
	Glandular Suprarenalis	Hepar
	Tuberculinum	Arsenicum
	Insecticide heel	Nux Vomica Inj.
	Cralonin	Engystol

9 For a more detailed exploration of homeopathy and the Seutermann protocols, see Shealy, *Energy Medicine* (pp. 185-91).

4th Week	Monday	Thursday
	Alpha Ketoglutarate	Succinyl Co-A
	Ubichinon	Antherachinon
	Thyroidea	Penicillin - Injeel
	Nosode Injeel	Tuberculinum
	Procainum	Tabacum
	Graphites	WWGinseng Comp.

5th Week	Monday	Thursday
	Succinic Acid	Fumaric Acid
	Chinhudron	Hydrochinon
	Placenta	Cerebrum
	Arsenicum	Lymphonyosot
	Psorinoheel	Pulsatilla
	Histamine	Hypericum

6th Week	Monday	Thursday
	Malic Acid	Oxaloacetic Acid
	Napthochinon	Parabenzochin Inj.
	Glandular Suprarenalis	Hepar
	Tuberculinum	Nosode Injeel
	Ranunculus	Sabal
	Ignatia	Medorrhinum

7th Week	Monday	Thursday
	Acetyl-Co-A	Glyoxal
	Ubichinon	Anthrachinon

Thyroidea

Glandular Suprarenalis

Arsenicum

Sulfonamide injeel

Sabadilla Injeel

Straphantus

Melliotus

Oleander

8th Week   Monday   Thursday

Methylglyoxal

Citric Acid

Anthrachinon

Chinhudron

Placenta

Cerebrum

Lymphomyosot

Nosode Injeel

Viscum Comp.

Arum

Rhododendron

Thuja

9th Week   Monday   Thursday

Cis Acontic Acid

Isocitrate

Hydrochinon

Napthochinon

Tetracycline

Hepar

Tuberculinum

Arsenicum

Tobacco Inj.

Tramajeel

NAD

Phosphorus

10th Week   Monday   Thursday

Oxalo Succinic Acid

Alphaketoglutarate

Parabenzochinon

Ubichinon

Thyroidea

Glandular Suprarenalis

Lymphomyosot

Tuberculinum

Vinum Bactense Injeel

Zeel

Acomitune

Arum Inj.

11th Week	Monday	Thursday
	Succinyl Co-A	Succinic Acid
	Anthnachinon	Chinhudron
	Placenta	Cerebrum
	Nosode Injeel	Lymphomyosot
	Causticum	Circulo Inj.
	Cactus Comp.	Galium
12th Week	Monday	Thursday
	Fumaric Acid	Malic Acid
	Hydrochinon	Ubichinon
	Staphylococcus	Thyroidea
	Tuberculinum	Gelsinium
	Cor	Procainum
	Kalmia	Sabadilla

The above list is based in Heel injectable liquid ampules (note that the FDA approves their oral use only). These can be obtained from BHI/Biological Homeopathic Industries, Inc. of Albuquerque, N. Mex. However, it may not be possible to order just a few ampules of each. For individual tablets of each, contact Celletech Ltd. Of Madison, Wisc. (see Appendix).

Other Herb Health Enhancers serve a variety of needs.

Agrimony: If your whole digestive system needs a lift, try out this herb, said to improve stomach, liver, kidney and gallbladder function.

Aloe: While great for healing burns and skin irritation when applied topically, orally it modulates the entire gastrointestinal system.

Angelica root: Traditional wisdom names this herb as a great heart strengthener, especially for those suffering from heart-related conditions.

Anise: This licorice-flavored herb can help prevent the accumulation of painful gas in the stomach and intestines

Arnica: The yellow flowers of this plant have powerful anti-inflammatory properties. Apply it to the skin to help reduce the pain and swelling of bruises, strains, and sprains.

Ashwagandha: Dose up to 2100 mg daily, improved when taken with black pepper. Its properties include:

> Reducing blood sugar.
> Decreasing growth of cancer.
> Decreasing cortisol.
> Reducing anxiety.
> Reducing depression.
> Increasing testosterone.
> Reducing body fat.
> Increasing muscle mass and strength.
> Reducing inflammation.
> Reducing cholesterol and triglycerides.
> Improving memory.

Aspalathus: This South African herb contains a number of antioxidants similar to those found in Bilberry. These can boost your eye health while giving you overall improved immune function.

Bacopa: Used in India for several thousand years, this flowering plant has been said to improve memory, learning, and cognition. Studies have shown that it can do little to improve your old memories but does have an effect on newly-acquired information, so start taking it sooner rather than later.

Berberine: Dose 500 mg 3 times a day. Its properties include:

Decreasing depression.
Acting as an antioxidant and anti-inflammatory.
Reducing growth of cancer.
Decreasing blood sugar.
Reducing fatty liver.
Improving immune system.
Improving congestive heart failure.

Bilberry: A relatively unknown but powerful antioxidant, bilberry has a number of positive health effects for the brain and heart. It can also help to protect the retina and improve range and clarity of vision.

Bilwa: Found in the sub-Himalayan forests, this fruit has been used in India to treat painful eye conditions like sties and conjunctivitis.

Brahmi: Use this Indian remedy to help boost your brain function and information retention.

Burnet: The leaves of this plant have been used for thousands of years in China. It helps heal burns and treats several skin conditions; it also reduces inflammation of hemorrhoids.

Burdock: Used all over the world, this herb helps combat hair loss, treats dandruff, and helps skin problems.

Calendula: Great for all-around skin care, this herb can treat everything from acne to chapped lips.

Catnip: Not just for cats, this common herb when eaten can help reduce anxiety and produce a mildly sedated effect.

Cat's Claw: While few definitive studies have been done, many believe this herb can reduce general inflammation and boost the immune system.

Cayenne: Containing capsicum, cayenne can help normalize blood pressure, increase the elasticity of blood vessels, and slow bleeding.

Celery Seed: Those having a little difficulty urinating may want to try this natural remedy, cited for its diuretic properties.

Chamomile: Generally known as a relaxing herb, chamomile tea can be a great way to wind down after a stressful day. Women have also used it to relieve menstrual cramps

Coriander: The seeds of the cilantro plant can help build and strengthen your circulatory system and make for a stronger, healthier heart.

Comfrey: Use the leaves and roots of this plant to soothe skin irritations and promote connective cell growth.

Cinnamon: If you're worried about the health of your circulatory system, consider adding a little cinnamon to your diet. Cinnamon has been shown to reduce blood sugar and help lower cholesterol.

Dandelion: Don't think of dandelion as just an annoying weed, since they can help control high blood pressure. Researchers think it works like many prescription medicines, decreasing blood volume and thereby blood pressure.

Devil's Claw: Native to southern Africa, this long-used remedy can be a helpful agent in reducing inflammation as well as back and neck pain.

Echinacea: Give your immune system a boost by taking some echinacea.

Ephedra: One of the oldest cultivated medicinal herbs, Ephedra is commonly used to help treat and prevent colds. It works by dilating the bronchial tubes through the release of adrenaline; it is especially useful to those suffering from allergies and asthma. Long-term usage can be harmful, however, so take it with care.

Fenugreek:

Lowers blood sugar.

Lowers cholesterol.

Improves lactation.

Prevents breast and colon cancer.

Decreases appetite.

Reduces risk of heart attack.

Prevents constipation and diarrhea.

Feverfew: Studies have confirmed that feverfew can help prevent and treat migraines. It works by reducing the amount of serotonin in the body and relaxing constricted blood vessels in the head.

Gamma Orizanol: Give this remedy a try to help calm an upset stomach.

Garlic: Garlic is a powerhouse when it comes to heart health. Regular usage has been shown to prevent cardiovascular disease and lower high blood pressure. In addition, studies suggest that it might help prevent cancer, kill bacteria, and even improve levels of t-cells in AIDS patients.

Gentian: This bitter herb has been used for generations to treat digestive problems. Its bitter taste stimulates the digestive system, making it easier to move food through your GI system problem-free.

Ginger: An upset stomach is never fun to deal with, but ginger may be the solution that you're looking for. Ginger helps slow the production of serotonin, a major factor in the nauseated feeling you get when you are motion sick or experiencing pregnancy sickness

Ginkgo Biloba: Ginkgo has been attached to many potential benefits, but perhaps one of the most significant is its ability to improve blood flow to the eyes especially in those suffering from macular degeneration. It can also be valuable to your ears as numerous studies have suggested it can help prevent tinnitus and inner ear disturbances as well as a number of other conditions.

Ginseng: Many people have heard of the herb ginseng, but few know of the numerous studies documenting its effects. These studies seem to suggest that its benefits include improved memory and other mental performance, immune system stimulation, and lowered cholesterol.

Goldenseal: Sties and conjunctivitis can be irritating and embarrassing conditions. Take some goldenseal to help reduce the inflammation associated with these conditions.

Holy Basil: Also known as tulsi, this herb is not usually used in cooking like its cousin, sweet basil; instead, it can help reduce the effects of stress on the body by inhibiting cortisol.

Guggul: Guggul is thought to bind to lipids in your gut so that you eliminate them before they enter your bloodstream, helping reduce your overall cholesterol. Dose 400 to 1000 mg daily. Guggul (or gugulipid):

> Reduces obesity.
> Is anti-inflammatory.
> Helps osteoarthritis.
> Reduces inflammation in colon.
> Assists thyroid function.
> Protects heart, liver, kidneys and brain.
> Has anti-cancer properties.

Gynostemia: Laboratory studies show this herb to have a direct effect on the circulatory system, strengthening the heart and helping wounds heal more quickly.

Hawthorn: The berries of this flowering shrub are great for the heart. They help open up the coronary arteries, lower blood pressure, and help slow a rapid heart rate. Users will see best effects after six months of taking the supplement.

Kava kava: By binding to brain receptors that promote relaxation, this herb can help anxiety.

Horse chestnut: Help prevent those unsightly varicose veins by taking some horse chestnut. Aescin and other compounds in the herb help bulk up weak capillaries and veins, making them less prone to swelling and pain.

Kudzu: Tired of killing all those brain cells with booze? This herb can help you to curb your craving by allowing alcohol to move more quickly to the part of the brain that tells you "enough is enough."

Licorice: You may love the taste of licorice but might not have known about its beneficial health effects. It can soothe and relax gastrointestinal tissues, helping ease the pain of ulcers and acid reflux; it has also been shown to help increase bile production.

Mahonia Grape Extract: The sun can have an immensely damaging effect on the eyes, but this herb can help reduce the impact of sun damage while strengthening the retina, slowing eye aging, and maintaining better overall eye health.

Marjoram: Great for general aches and pains, this common herb can be even more effective when combined with chamomile or gentian.

Meadowsweet: The roots of meadowsweet contain many of the chemicals used to make aspirin; when chewed, it can prove a helpful remedy for headaches.

Milk Thistle: Give your liver some help filtering out all those toxins by taking some milk thistle. As demonstrated in testing done at radiology tech schools, it can help improve the regeneration of liver tissue and regulate liver function.

Motherwort: This plant has a long history of use and contains the alkaloid leonurine, which can have a relaxing effect on smooth muscles like those found in the heart.

Mullein flower: This flowering plant acts as a natural bactericide; when condensed to oil form, it offers a natural treatment for ear infection.

Plantain leaf: Because of its many soothing properties, this plant is a popular remedy for cuts, skin infections, and chronic skin problems.

Peppermint Oil: A little dab of peppermint oil will help relax the smooth muscles of your colon, stopping the cramps and constipation that can be common symptoms of irritable bowel syndrome. Peppermint tea is excellent for digestion.

Red Clover: If you've "tried everything" to get rid of acne, you might give this natural acne and skin clearing remedy a try.

Rose Hips: These small berries serve a dual purpose, helping reduce bladder infections and fight constipation.

Sage: As modern research has shown, this herb *can* actually help make you "sage" by improving memory while reducing inflammation.

Sassafras Leaf: Said to purify and cleanse the body, this plant can help control acne.

Senna: If you're feeling constipated, this herb works as a natural laxative.

St. John's Wort: Those with mild to moderate depression may find some relief with this herb. Numerous studies have shown that, in many cases, it can be as effective as some prescription drugs.

Solomon's Seal Root: Make a wash out of this plant to help control skin problems and blemishes.

Spikenard: Treat acne, pimples, blackheads, and rashes with this inflammation-fighting herb.

Suma: This Amazon rainforest plant can help normalize body systems and reduce the effects of stress.

Thyme: Many use thyme in their cooking without being aware that it can help fight infection, reduce the pain of migraines, and clear out the lungs.

Uva Ursi: This herb is a remedy for bladder irritation.

Valerian: Lull your body into a restful sleep with this natural remedy. Replacing prescription medications, valerian has been shown to be effective while eliminating the more harmful side effects of sleeping pills.

Willow Bark: A component of aspirin, willow bark can naturally reduce minor aches and pains.

Witch Hazel: Those suffering from hemorrhoids will appreciate the anti-inflammatory properties of this herb.

Wood Betony: This attractive woodland plant can be used to reduce the pain associated with headaches.

3. Reducing Stress: "It's not what you're eating, it's what's eating you …"

In *The Creation of Health: The Emotional, Psychological, and Spiritual Responses that Promote Health and*

Healing, Dr. Shealy's co-author, Caroline Myss, identified eight dysfunctional patterns of behavior and attitude, each stress-related, and each leading to illness.[10] The first pattern "involves the presence of unresolved or deeply consuming emotional, psychological or spiritual stress within a person's life" (p. 8). Divorce or death of a spouse or child can trigger this pattern, though its root cause can reach back to childhood and one's "feeling of rejection or inadequacy" (p. 8).

The second dysfunctional pattern "relates to the degree of control that negative belief patterns have upon a person's reality" (p. 8). "Each of us," writes Myss, "is a complex system of positive and negative beliefs, attitudes and experiences," and "because what we believe is intimately connected to our emotions, our beliefs influence our emotional response to life" (p. 8). Hence, people who fall ill "tend to have belief patterns that are disempowering," which "override the influence of whatever positive attitudes exist." Thus "an individual may be educated and talented and give the appearance of having all things working in his or her favor," while "underneath that illusion, that person may have such low self-esteem that he or she feels unworthy of success" (pp. 8-9).

The third pattern of dysfunction "is the inability to give and/or receive love" (Myss, p. 9). People's lives "revolve around love, and when stressful experiences in relationships exist, the physical body can easily break down in response. A person who lives a life devoid of love

---

10 See Shealy and Myss, *The Creation of Health: The Emotional, Psychological, and Spiritual Responses that Promote Health and Healing* (New York: Three Rivers Press, 2009).

or of any degree of human warmth is a prime candidate for disease" (p. 9).

The fourth pattern "is lack of humor and the inability to distinguish serious concerns from the lesser issues of life" (Myss, p. 9). The key, writes Myss, is "learning how to let go of the lesser stuff in order to avoid problems such as high blood pressure, migraines or ulcers. Laughter is extremely healing" (p. 9). Amen! Learning "to let go" is part of the Shealy-Sorin protocol for stress-reduction in life.

The fifth pattern "is how effectively one exercises the power of choice in terms of holding dominion over the movement and activities of their own life" (Myss, p. 10). This needs some explaining. "Holding dominion," she writes, "does not mean always getting one's own way. It means being able to participate in the natural give and take of life, to be flexible, to respond to the needs of others and to reach for what you need from a position of inner strength and confidence" (p. 10). The health implications here are real, indeed:

> Every person must feel that he or she has a choice in the matters of his or her own life. When the dynamic of choice is violated or interfered with, a person's emotional response can often lead to the development of disease. This is because the individual's response to a violation of choice will be filled with anger, hostility, fear and rage. (Myss, p. 10)

The sixth pattern "concerns how well a person has attended to the needs of the physical body itself" (Myss, p. 10). Of course we agree. In particular, we appreciate the emphasis she places on the different stresses—emotional, physical, and chemical—that impact the body: "Nutrition, exercise, the impact of drugs or alcohol, as well as a person's genetic makeup, provide the foundation for the quality of health. How well an individual attends to the emotional, physical and chemical stresses of life is very strongly connected to the degree of vigor and stamina in the physical body itself" (pp. 10-11).

The seventh pattern "relates to the 'existential vacuum' or the suffering that accompanies the absence or loss of meaning in one's life" (Myss, p. 11). While this "loss of meaning" is felt by the individual, it's a marker of a larger, cultural crisis: Modernity itself—life in the 21st century—is experienced as an existential crisis. *Why* death? *Why* suffering? *Why* injustice? *Why* poverty? *Why* war? *Why* crime? Focusing specifically on 21st century crises, we ask ourselves: *Why* the failure of antibiotics? *Why* the massive extermination of planetary species? *Why* the poisoning of our ecosystem? *Why* the warming climate and rising seas? *Why* the seeming inevitability of environmental collapse? "The lost soul," writes Myss, "is very susceptible to illness, primarily because a life devoid of meaning often leads to despair, depression and feelings of worthlessness. The physical body is strongly affected when one's state of mind and emotions are consumed with the suffering that comes from feelings of emptiness" (p. 11). She adds, "this is a frequent condition reported by people who are ill" (p. 11). She's right, though we'd add that "the modern condition" is grounded in despair—or, more precisely, in an insane cycle of euphoric consumption (of material goods, entertainments, drugs and other distractions) alternating with feelings of despair. Our task is to turn clinical depression and private despair into the more humane, therapeutic process of grieving, since grief is our native human response to loss. And we have lost a great deal: Whole planetary species are gone (with many, many more threatened with extinction); the ways we once gathered and interacted socially have been lost to "social distancing in an age of viral pandemic. Older readers will attest to the fact that "this is not the world we grew up in," even if the warning signs were there all along, staring us in the face. Let's not be Pollyannas and pretend that the modern "existential vacuum" can be willed away or changed by mere mood. No: Let's learn to grieve for what we've lost, since peace and acceptance lie on the other side of grief, whereas depression and despair know no end.

The eighth pattern "is the tendency toward denial. Tremendous inner stress is created from the inability to face the challenges of one's life and neither to acknowledge nor consciously recognize what it is that is not working in one's life" (Myss, p. 11). It's precisely this habit of denial that we're seeking to counter in the paragraph above. The first step in solving depression is to admit that you're depressed. Then, you need the courage *to name* your depression and its causes, which may be physical, or social, or political, or familial, or economic, or ecological. "Much of this stress," Myss continues, "is created as a result of choosing to block one's own intuition or awareness in order to allow certain situations to continue without addressing the deeper problems that exist" (p. 11). Again, we say amen.

Let's summarize Prof. Myss's patterns of dysfunctional attitude, belief, and behavior that lead to mental and physical illness. These are as follows:

Unresolved emotional, psychological,
or spiritual stress.
The control that negative belief patterns have
upon a person's reality.
The inability to give and/or receive love.
Lack of humor (and an inability to let go of the
"lesser stuff").
Loss of a sense of choice in "holding dominion" over
one's life.
Failure to attend to the needs of the body.
Existential despair over the loss of meaning in life.
The tendency toward denial (which blocks one's
powers of intuition).

Dealing with Negative Emotions: Moving from internal will to transcendence.

Emotions (positive or negative) are feelings that are tied to (and, hence, are responsive to) our attitudes/

beliefs; they send messages that tell us when a situation feels good/safe/okay or threatening/uncomfortable/unsafe/not okay. We argue that, while there are many names for these, there are in fact four negative emotions: anger, guilt, depression, and anxiety. All other negative emotions are aspects of these four. Such feelings as frustration, disappointment, etc. are synonyms for anger, guilt, depression, and anxiety. And all negative emotions are a reaction to fear of loss—to loss of life, of health, of financial security, of love, of moral values, or of existential meaning.

Anger, like all negative, stressful emotions, is one reaction to fear. Often it is fear of loss of love (approval, acceptance, social security, etc.). But anger may come from fear of loss of money (job, financial security, etc.) or of moral integrity (i.e., a righteous indignation that someone else is doing something "wrong"). Rarely is anger a reaction to fear of illness or death. Anger is the most natural reaction to a perceived threat. It is a survival instinct, tied to the body's "fight or flight" response. But note that anger, in itself, is not a solution to stress.

Guilt is anger with self, a feeling that one has not lived up to one's potential or expectations. Note that conscience is an expression of conscientiousness: We should strive to live in accordance with our moral values and, when we fall short, that "warning voice" inside can and should spur us on to correct our attitudes and behaviors. Guilt, however, typically involves some perceived inadequacy and low self-esteem. Though often equated with that internal "voice of conscience," guilt is in fact a mode of conditioning by parents especially, though other family members as well as teachers and friends contribute their share. When we accept and internalize the expectations of others, we set ourselves up to feel guilt—and guilt never solves anything. Certainly, it never resolves one's sense of inadequacy or low self-esteem. In fact, guilt feeds into the next negative emotion: depression.

Depression has many facets—emotional, social, spiritual, existential. As an emotion, it's marked by the loss of joy in life. In many respects, it marks the "triumph" of low self-esteem, since it implies powerlessness over one's life and its situations. Who, after all, would choose depression if he or she had a choice or a chance to change? This sense of powerlessness leads to a sense of hopelessness, which, at its lowest point, leads one into a trough of despair. Like other negative emotions, depression never solves one's problems but only makes one's situation worse—especially since this emotion, being a form of "passive aggression" *against the self*, gives up even on the possibility of change.

Anxiety is another word for fear that has become vague and generalized—lacking in a specific object. When FDR declared, nobly, "We have nothing to fear, but fear itself," it was the anxiety of the nation he was trying to calm. People with anger-management problems are at least occasionally anger-free; similarly, guilt comes and goes. Much like depression, however, anxiety can become a constant, debilitating presence—as well as a self-fulfilling prophecy. If your fear lacks an object or nameable cause, *it will most surely find one!*

The solution to all emotional distress is a double-barreled dose of spiritual discipline and common sense. Remember your God-given reason and your intuition! And remember to use them together, allowing your intuition to bolster reason, and vice versa. Treat these as your left and right hands and learn to be ambidextrous. (We've known many people good at one but not the other: Intuition without reason sees the forest but neglects the trees, whereas reason without intuition sees the trees—the material world—only.) Wisdom demands both: Call no one wise who lacks either spiritual discipline or common sense.[11] Common sense tells us that, no matter what the cause of the distress, no matter what the fear or emotional reaction, there is a limit to what is possible in life. Take the object of your anger, for example, and view it under the light of reason. Do a realistic appraisal of your options—of what you can actually do to correct, stop, or change the perceived problem. Can you stop or change it by calm discussion? What good would a temper tantrum do? Would writing a letter or fighting or going to court do any good? If you *can* stop or change the situation, are you

---

11 In *Medical Intuition: Awakening to Wholeness* (Virginia Beach, VA: A.R.E. Press, 2010), Shealy quotes German theologian, Adolf Lasson (1832-1917): "'The essence of mysticism is the assertion of an intuition that transcends the temporal categories of the understanding, relying on speculative reason. Rationalism cannot conduct us to the essence of things; we therefore need intellectual vision.' He is calling intellectual vision here actually a form of intuition" (p. 71). The point: *reason and intuition need each other.*

willing to put forth the energy and effort? Is it *worth* the effort? There are numerous situations which you may not like and which are potentially changeable, but how many windmills can you tilt?

If you cannot or choose not to change the situation, can you escape it? Can you detach from it and divorce it with joy, knowing you will no longer have to live with an intolerable situation? If you can divorce the problem, are you *willing* to divorce it? Does the bad in the situation outweigh the good? Or do the good aspects of the situation outweigh the bad? Make a list of the positives and the negatives and weigh each list on a scale of 1 to 10. Be elaborate and complete in your listing. If you decide that divorce is best, will you proceed without guilt, allowing yourself to be happy—indeed, joyous—knowing that you don't have to put up with the bad anymore?

If you cannot or choose not to change the situation, and you cannot or choose not to divorce it, then you have one further option: to accept and forgive. Think back to your close friendships and relationships: Surely you've had more than a few opportunities to exercise forgiveness, overlooking inadequacies, faults, and idiosyncratic behaviors. In the situation you're facing, are you willing to make friends with it, to be generous and forgiving?[12]

_____

12 An inability to forgive and to tolerate differences is a common cause of anger and anxiety, which are foundations for depression. The Native American philosophy of not criticizing someone "until you have walked in their moccasins" applies here: It teaches us to be accepting of others' choices and actions, just as Christ declared, "let him who is without sin cast the first stone" (John 8.3).

Let's tap into your intuition now and ask the "whole person"—body, mind, spirit—to aid in your decision-making. Don't just *think* the solution: Truly *feel* it, as well. Enter a state of deep relaxation and become attuned to your subtle body feelings. Then ask yourself which feels better: Changing/stopping the situation? Divorcing with joy? Or accepting and forgiving? None of these options may feel perfect, but you can find your personal best solution by joining logic to intuition. Ultimately, *you* are responsible for your anger, guilt, depression, and anxiety. So ask yourself:

Does my anger (guilt, depression, anxiety) make me feel good?

Can I solve the problem by being upset?

Do I have a right to insist that someone or something else change for my benefit?

Am I perfect? Can I expect perfection from others?

Can I correct the problem by being upset?

Do I enjoy being upset?

Am I willing to put forth the effort to overcome my upset?

Do I want to be: forgiving; tolerant; serene—at peace?

Do I consider forgiveness, tolerance, serenity to be spiritual goals?

Am I willing to be good to myself and others by

being forgiving, tolerant, serene?
Do I want to do good to others? Do I want to do
good to myself?
Am I willing to live the Golden Rule?

Dealing with negative emotions (anger, guilt, depression, anxiety) requires the spiritual discipline of living the Golden Rule: Doing until others as you wish to have done to you. When you train yourself to live this transcendent principle, you will:

Analyze each situation carefully.

Discern what is acceptable or unacceptable.

Change those unacceptable situations which you can and choose to change.

Detach from those situations which you cannot or choose not to change (divorce or accept/forgive).

Become (and remain) nonjudgmental.

Have no need to know why.

Be at peace with everything that you cannot or choose not to change.

Only practice, practice, practice will allow you to experience and live these principles of spiritual discipline. Ideally, you will train yourself to make such decisions rapidly, almost instantly, in order to live the Golden Rule and to be at peace with yourself and with life. In this way, spiritual discipline infuses one's daily activities: As the Christian mystic, Evelyn Underhill

(1875-1941) once said, the spiritual life is "the attitude you hold in your mind when you are down on your knees scrubbing the steps." And attitude determines your emotions. If your attitude is a positive one of acceptance, serenity, and love, then your emotions will be joyous, blissful even. If your attitude is a negative one of fear or suspicion, you'll be giving yourself over to anger, guilt, depression, anxiety. Which of these sets of feelings do you prefer? The choice is yours. The solution is yours. The responsibility is yours.

At the clinic, we give out "Stress Management Pocket Cards," aimed at helping our clients make decisions and take actions to reduce daily stress. They're laminated and about the size of a credit card, so they're easy to carry around and consult. The card, front and back, is included on the next page.

This card is the summary of our life philosophy and approach to stress. If something is not right or is a concern, and if you can do something about it in the present moment, then go ahead and do what you are willing to do to make things better. If you are not able or willing to do something about it and it's still concerning you, then only two healthy choices are recommended:

Detach: Let go of those things that you are not able or willing to fight.

Go for sainthood: Forgive, let go, and leave those things simply to be.

Otherwise, spending your precious time and energy on things that you cannot or will not take positive action will only lead to chronic illness.

Urban Lifestyle: Contributing to stress.

We've become a nation of city dwellers. There are positives and negatives to the modern urban lifestyle. We've been discussing how best to live: Does it matter *where* you live? A recent *USA Today* article, "25 of the most dangerous cities in America,"[13] presents some sobering statistics on violent crime—murder, manslaughter, rape,

---

13 "25 of the most dangerous cities in America," *USA Today*, August 14, 2019 (https://www.usatoday.com/picture-gallery/travel/experience/america/2018/10/17/25-most-dangerous-cities-america/1669467002/), accessed 1 March 2020. Crimes statistics are given for the year 2017.

armed robbery, assault—per 100,000 population. Here's the "top 25" in this dubious category: 25. Beaumont, TX (1,063); 24. Chattanooga, TN (1,066), 23. Hartford, CT (1,093); 22. Houston, TX (1,095); 21. Chicago, IL (1,099); 20. Minneapolis, MN (1,101); 19. New Orleans, LA (1,121); 18. Lansing, MI (1,136); 17. Nashville, TN (1,138); 16. Anchorage, AK (1,203); 15. San Bernadino, CA (1,291); 14. Oakland, CA (1,299); 13. Indianapolis, IN (1,334); 12. Springfield, MO (1,339); 11. Albuquerque, NM (1,369); 10. Stockton, CA (1,415); 9. Cleveland, OH (1,557); 8. Rockford, IL (1,588); 7. Milwaukee, WI (1,597); 6. Little Rock, AR (1,634); 5. Kansas City, MO (1,724); 4. Memphis, TN (2,003); 3. Baltimore, MD (2,027); 2. Detroit, MI (2,057); 1. St. Louis, MO (2,082). Of course the incidents of crime increases stress; in which case, who'd want to live in a city?

Wholeness: Georgianne Ginder on "thoughts after a recent American Holistic Nurses Association meeting." She writes, "This was after the banquet and dancing on the eve of the last day":

> I felt as I watched the rhythm of the wholeness, which was music, which was heartbeat, which was connection, which was joy, which was trust, which surrounded and grounded and extolled and connected ... which was and is life itself ... I observed that even those who were not able to join the circle of dance were dancing nonetheless—all souls moving

and swaying. A gentleman in a wheeled chair
and others perhaps too shy or having pain and
so on ... included themselves and were included
nonetheless. I, sadly, grew weary and pained and
departed early. I was returning (hobbling actually
to my hotel-sanctuary) after the banquet and the
dancing. And, as it so very often happens when the
world of words flow, these words came to me: "the
music plays and someone prays."

Soon I heard footsteps behind me. It was dusk
and rain was beginning to fall and I had spied groups of
persons standing in the shadows as I passed .... Was I
safe? I felt the slightest clutch, being prone to all sorts of
scenarios happening simultaneously all the time ... but I
asked for I asked God's abiding protection and grace as I
caned my way toward my resting place. I use a cane now
for support and balance after the foot reconstruction, so I
felt more vulnerable than usual.

But I willed myself not to be afraid. And I felt secure
and protected for I had asked! Leaning, as I was, and
always am, upon the everlasting arms ....

Later on, I pondered once more on holistic
"health"—being and living whole and always healed,
which is/was the charge of those who attended this

beautiful forceful field of caring, opportunity, and sharing. I recalled what Dr. Edward Gabrielle had shared at the close of the session at the Smithsonian conference about Health, Wellness and Martin Luther King: The ancient Latin word *salvus*—meaning "safe," "sound," "alive," "unharmed," and "well"—gave us the English word "salvation." And so it was that I was safe and sound and well. And whole:

> The music plays ...
> Then someone sways
> As someone prays
>
> All ways
> All days
> Always
> Someone prays
>   (Someone's praise)
>
> Always—
> The music plays ...

DNA, Methylation, and Life Expectancy: Where the Shealy-Sorin Protocol all comes together...

Happy people live longer: That's a fact. At the Shealy-Sorin wellness Institute, we're developing protocols to give people back this "genetic birthright"—a century of life well-lived. Our DNA indicates that we're programmed genetically to live 100 years, but the average American achieves only 78% of that potential. This isn't due entirely to lack of conscientiousness. Even with good health habits, our telomeres—the tips of our DNA—shrink 1% each year.[14] Our genetic makeup is "preprogrammed" at conception, and yet our genes, paradoxically, are epigenetic—that is, they're influenced by external factors, including stress (and our reaction to stress), nutrition, the environment, etc. And severe adverse influences can affect genes many generations later.

The habits of a mother during pregnancy affect the baby significantly, so that an alcoholic or smoking or obese mother will adversely affect the baby, both genetically and epigenetically. Also, the ability of the mother to handle the methyl transfer is highly genetic. In the biochemical processes of methylation, methyl donors are as important as oxygen. The ability to transfer methyl depends on the sulfur molecule (such as MSM) as well as on choline, trimethyl glycine, folic acid, and vitamin B12. All of these require the essential vitamins, amino acids, omega 3 fatty acids, and minerals.

Chronic stress depletes us of these essential methyl donors, which then shorten our DNA telomeres. This is

---

14 See M. E. Levine et al., "An epigenetic biomarker of aging for lifespan and healthspan," *Aging* 10.4 (2018): 573-591. Telomeres are the tips of each DNA strand. DNA—Deoxyribonucleic acid—is a complex molecule composed of two chains that coil around each other, forming that famous "double helix" that you've surely heard of (and may have studied in school). As the essential building block of life on planet Earth, it carries genetic instructions for the development, functioning, growth, and reproduction of all known organisms.

a major reason why stress ages people prematurely and leads to chronic physical and mental fatigue. Higher levels of basic multivitamins and of folic acid are associated with longer telomeres. Homocysteine is a strongly genetically-influenced contributor to every aspect of metabolism. There is considerable evidence that maintaining a homocysteine level of 7.5 (and no higher) is essential for increased longevity and prevention of many diseases. And yet labs wrongly list the upper limit of homocysteine as 11 to 14. Higher levels of homocysteine lead to shorter DNA telomeres and increased atherosclerosis. Folic acid and methyl folate is crucial to keeping homocysteine levels low.

Antioxidants are needed to decrease inflammation and reduce free-radical damage to telomeres—not to mention the role of antioxidants in reducing risks of cancer. Also, at least 80% of Americans are low in intracellular magnesium. Low levels of intracellular magnesium are associated with shorter DNA telomeres. Hence, magnesium supplementation is essential for DNA repair and replication.

Both zinc and copper are essential for telomere health. A novel antioxidant that contains zinc is carnosine, which has been shown to slow the rate of telomere depletion in human fibroblast cells while extending their longevity. Carnosine is also a major brain antioxidant, making it a great stress management nutrient. Numerous antioxidants are likely to help protect and repair DNA. Carnosine, tocotrienols, vitamin D3, and vitamin C are all essential for telomere health. Excess weight (and especially obesity) leads to telomere shortening. Clinically, it has been shown that individuals with the highest levels of vitamin D have longer telomeres. Other antioxidants—such as quercetin, green tea, curcumin, and resveratrol—also assist in DNA protection and repair. But do you see how big a role the Shealy-Sorin "basic essentials" play in telomere length and life expectancy? And do you see how stresses of all sort—physical, emotional, environmental—contribute to DNA damage, thereby shortening life? We began this book with a lay-sermon on conscientiousness. Do you see how personality traits contribute to life choices which can either lengthen or shorten one's life?

Yes, smoking "kills," poor nutrition "kills," lack of exercise "kills." Cancers, diabetes, and hypertension are implicated in these behaviors. But DNA telomere length provides a measurable marker of *quality* as well as of length of life. Stress of all kinds leads to increasingly shorter telomeres. People with hypertension, diabetes, coronary artery disease, Parkinsonism, Alzheimer's, and cancer have shorter telomeres. Children born to parents with premature coronary artery disease have shorter telomeres. (They start life at a genetic disadvantage, in other words.) In contrast, individuals with a positive personality have longer telomeres. Telomeres are significantly longer in people of higher socioeconomic status. At birth, there is no difference in telomere length between women and men; but women in adulthood have longer telomeres than men. (And women have a longer life expectancy, right? Are you beginning to see the pattern?)

Since the days of Albert Einstein (1879-1955), scientists have long sought for a Grand Unified Theory, a model of the material world and its forces (electromagnetic and subatomic) that could "hold everything together" and, in effect, "explain everything" *without exception and contradiction.* Though models have been proposed, quantum physics has yet to settle on its "Theory of Everything." Of course, holistic medicine seeks "the whole" in holism. And that, dear reader, is what we have unveiled in this book: a Grand Unified Theory of holistic health that draws on all facets of the human creature—genetic, neurochemical, metabolic, reproductive, nutritional, behavioral, social, spiritual, environmental— in order to restore a happy, healthy century-long lifespan to clients. We make this bold claim, because we have demonstrated clinically in fifty test cases that it's possible for adults of average health *to increase their telomere length* by 3.5% each year—in effect reversing the aging process. Bioelectric enhancement is key to increasing longevity, and the Shealy-Sorin protocol includes the following:

• Sitting or lying one hour daily under a copper pyramid activated by a Tesla coil.

• Lying on a RejuvaMatrix mattress (with embedded Tesla coil) one hour each night.

• Stimulating the "Sacred Rings" of Fire, Earth and Crystal each day with the SheLi TENS using 52 to 78 GHz frequencies.

• Applying Shealy Fire, Earth, and Crystal Bliss oils daily.

Don't let the seeming strangeness of the above list daunt you; the pages following will explain. (For discussion of the "Sacred Rings" and Bliss oils, you'll need to wait until Chapter 4.)

Everything discussed so far fits into this holistic model, including the personality traits of common sense and conscientiousness. Of course the basics still apply: You can't live a long, healthy life unless you maintain healthy weight, avoid tobacco, eat five or more servings of veggies and fruits daily, exercise thirty minutes at least five days a week, and sleep 7-8 hours each night. But it's time now to add energy medicine.

4. Energy Medicine for the 21st Century

Of all Dr. Shealy's medical innovations, it's his contributions to energy medicine that have earned him international fame. Beginning in the early 1960's, Shealy introduced electroacupuncture, the use of electrical activation of acupuncture needles. Then he introduced spinal cord stimulation, which is still used worldwide for treatment of otherwise intractable pain. This led to his development of Transcutaneous Electrical Nerve Stimulation (TENS), still used worldwide for local pain. In 1976, he introduced Cranial Electrical Stimulation for treatment of depression, anxiety, insomnia, and jet lag. All of these are safe, except for those with an implanted electrical device (such as a pacemaker) or in pregnancy.

In the 1990s, Shealy introduced RejuvaMatrix Solar

Homeopathy, a therapeutic mattress whose modified Tesla coil produces 52 to 78 GHz at one billionth of a watt per cm square, in order to rejuvenate human DNA telomeres and overall health and longevity. This, too, is safe except for those with an implanted electrical device or in pregnancy.

Who was Georges Lakhovsky? Most readers will have heard of Nikola Tesla, but what of the Belarusian-French Georges Lakhovsky (1869-1942)? In 1925, he developed the Multiple Wave Oscillator—in effect, a powerful modified Tesla coil useful in treating cancer. The Lakhovsky coil was a common feature in American hospitals through the beginning of World War II. Lakhovsky himself declared a high cure rate for some cancers—as high as 98%. Inexplicably, the instrument was removed from American hospitals soon after his death and eventually banned altogether. But good ideas get reborn: The coil accompanying the RejuvaMatrix mattress is a modern version of the Lakhovsky Multiple Wave Oscillator. As noted, we recommend this device for general health and longevity. It also serves as an adjunct to numerous holistic, energy-based treatments, including viral infections and cancer.

There's always a moral to this sort of story. The Third Party—that unholy alliance of government agencies, mainstream medicine, and the pharmaceutical industry, which we excoriated in Chapter 1—has actively suppressed bioenergetic treatments, along with their practitioners and inventors. ("Don't I know it!" says Dr. Shealy, half-laughing, half-sighing.) Some of the work being done today rests in the recovery and reinvention of what has been lost through over-regulation and downright repression.

In 2015, the Shealy-Sorin Chakra-Sweep PEMF was introduced, with frequencies of 5.83 to 56.81 Hz. This device has a power field of three to four feet in all directions, allowing the body's cells to reset to the most essential electrical rhythm of -70 mV, crucial for normal function. The Chakra-Sweep PEMF has been found useful in relieving most types of pain; it improves blood-oxygenation levels in those with lung disease; it reduces blood pressure; and it aids in reducing anxiety, depression, insomnia, and addiction cravings. This device, too, is safe except for those with an implanted electrical device or in pregnancy. Descriptions of these and other Shealy-Sorin devices follow.

The Shealy-Sorin Autogenic Training System: Taking control of body, mind, and spirit.

For more than a century, the concept of self-regulation has been scientifically studied. In Chapter 1, we cited Dr. Schultz's research in Autogenic Training, which demonstrated that 80% of stress-related illness could be managed successfully with AT. In the early 1970's, Dr. Elmer Green introduced biofeedback training, using feedback from EEG, galvanic skin temperature, and EMG to assist patients in a wide variety of chronic illnesses, including migraine and hypertension.

In 1977, Dr. Shealy introduced Biogenics, which has been of great benefit in thousands of patients with chronic pain and depression. Using biofeedback, the Biogenics system assists individuals in controlling specific body sensations and muscle tension, as well as in releasing past trauma. Biogenics optimizes brain, mind, body, and spirit health. There are over 50 mp3s of Biogenics exercises, many amplified with health-enhancing music and sound frequencies. Topics include the following:

Be Here Now: Staying in present time.

Belief in Self: Using biofeedback as proof that the mind leads the body (and can heal the body).

Relaxation: Using breathe to control pain and calm the mind and body.

Talk to the Body & Mind: Autogenic Training with organ-specific affirmations.

Progressive Relaxation: Tensing to relax (shown by Edmund Jacobson to help 80% of patients with chronic diseases).

Love it: Learning to accept one's body and its challenges.

Collect and Release: Useful for pain control.

Circulate Electrical Energy: An exercise in regulating the piezoelectric aspects of the body.

Breathing Through the Skin: A superb exercise in pain control.

Expanding Your Electromagnetic Field: An exercise in "the Christos effect" for releasing past trauma.

Balancing Emotions: Over a dozen Gestalt and related exercises.

Past Life.

Self-Image.

Age Regression.

Zen Practice.

Spiritual attunement.

Meeting Your Soul.

Meeting Your Personal Angel.

Vibrational Music and Samvit Sound Technology: Music and sound have been used for millennia to assist healing and well-being. In 1988, using BETAR to enhance physical sensation of the music, Shealy found great additional benefit in depression, anxiety and pain. Today vibratory music is used with Biogenics to enhance success.

The Shealy-Sorin Autogenic Training System also comes with Samvit Sound Technology, which works with the brain via therapeutic frequencies that foster relaxation, healthful functioning of the limbic system (wellspring of emotions and memories), spiritual insight, and heightened mental awareness—that feeling of being "in the zone."

Biogenics AT exercises are essential for those with stress-related conditions. Just as important, they help reduce stress *before* it develops into full-blown medical/emotional problems. As noted in Chapter 1, people should make AT exercises a daily practice in immunization/inoculation starting in childhood—as early as age five.

To give a taste of AT exercises, several examples (focusing on pain control) follow. (For the actual scripts, you'll need to listen to the mp3s available at the Wellness Institute.)

Collect and Release: Once you have practiced this adequately, you can collect all pain from a given area. Practice breathing in and collecting, as with a gentle vacuum cleaner, all sensations:

From your feet.

From your legs.

From your buttocks and pelvis.

From your abdomen and low back.

From your entire chest.

From your shoulders, arm and hands.

From your neck.

From your entire head.

From toes to head.

Repeat this exercise, returning to focus on each area twice.

Breathing Through the Skin: Focusing your attention, imagine you are breathing through the skin of your right hand, in and back out. With sufficient practice, you can make your right hand totally numb! Once you have mastered this exercise, you can do the same with the left hand—and then with any area of pain.

Expanding Your Electromagnetic Field: Everything in your body is electrical and electricity creates magnetism. Relax and imagine that you are creating a one-inch electromagnetic field (EMF)—an aura capsule one inch in diameter—

> Surrounding your feet.
> Surrounding your legs.
> Surrounding your pelvis.
> Surrounding your abdomen and lower back.
> Surrounding your entire chest.
> Surrounding your shoulders, arms and hands.
> Surrounding your neck and entire head.

Then return to your feet and imagine the EMF field is expanding to twelve inches in diameter. Slowly expand the 12-inch EMF:

> Surrounding your feet.
> Surrounding your legs.
> Surrounding your pelvis.
> Surrounding your abdomen and lower back.
> Surrounding your entire chest.
> Surrounding your shoulders, arms and hands.
> Surrounding your neck and entire head.

Once in this state, you'll note that your mind is alert but your body feels absent or floating in space, with no physical sensations or pain. Stay in this state for at least ten minutes and learn to use it to get rid of any pain!

For further directions in self-regulation, follow the protocol outlined in Shealy's bestselling book, *90 Days to Self-Health.*[15] Practice deep relaxation at least thirty minutes daily, avoid negative news, violent movies, and if weather allows, replace television with lounging and walking outside—appreciate nature and the divine! And do these:

Practice Biogenics AT exercises.
Use the Shealy RelaxMate if you cannot relax quickly and easily.
Apply Shealy Fire and Air Bliss Oils twice per day.
Double the daily dose of magnesium lotion/spray.

If not much improved in four weeks, add the following:

• Read and practice *30 days to Self-Health* along with Biogenics audio exercises.
• Fisher-Wallace cranial stimulator transcranial one hour each morning.

---

15 Visitors to the Institute's website (www.ShealyWellness.com) who sign up for the mailing list can receive an e-book version free of charge.

• Shealy-Sorin RelaxMate II an hour before bedtime and 20 to 60 minutes anytime during the day.
• Shealy-Sorin Chakra Sweep Gamma PEMF 2 hours transcranially (over baseball cap) daily.
• A series of ten Myer's cocktail IVs with Magnesium and 75 to 100 grams of vitamin C.

The Shealy RelaxMate: It has been known since the discovery of EEG in the 1920s that the brain functions at different frequencies.

DELTA: 1 to 3 cycles per second—deep relaxation, especially just before sleep

THETA: 4 to 7 cycles per second—relaxation and creative visualization

ALPHA: 8 to 12 cycles per second—relaxation with little imagery

BETA: 13-23 cycles per second—alert listening, learning receiving.

HIGH BETA: 24-30 cycles per second—anxiety

GAMMA: 31-100 cycles per second.

The Shealy RelaxMate is an optical device (resembling sunglasses) that provides visual flickers of red or blue (or mixtures of red and blue) at 1 to 7 Hz, the optimal frequencies for relaxation: 95% of individuals find themselves more relaxed using these frequencies, with a majority preferring 1 to 3 Hz. This Hz range is useful in reducing anxiety and depression and in preparation for sleep. 40 Hz is the optimal "in the zone" state for happiness, creativity, peace and memory, productivity, energy, intellect, efficacy, recall, focus, and overall health. Interestingly, at 40 Hz, light is no longer visible as a frequency flicker but instead appears as a steady light. Optimal Gamma frequency is achieved by people well-practiced in meditation; as a modality of energy medicine, it is most effectively produced by the Shealy-Sorin Chakra Sweep Gamma PEMF.

SheLi TENS Unit: With its electrodes placed above and below a site of pain (or on either side of the pain), the SheLi TENS Unit remains one of the most common, safe, and effective tools for pain control. TENS therapy works by stimulating electrically the beta sensory fibers that carry only touch and vibratory sensations and which block pain fiber input. It gives off a pleasant tingling sensation and should be used a minimum of one hour (and up to 24 hours if needed). The major contraindication is an implanted electrical device, such as a pacemaker.

The Eight Pain-Relieving TENS Combos: If local relief is not achieved, then there are several other placements that may provide total body pain relief. A skilled acupuncturist will recognize the following notation as meridian points. Many of the CAM modalities described in this book adapt traditional Eastern acupuncture/meridian therapy to 21ˢᵗ century bioelectric technologies; the TENS combos are a case in point.

MH 6: On the palmar aspect of the forearm, 2 cun above the transverse crease of the wrist.

TH 5: 2 cun proximal to the dorsal wrist crease between the radius and ulna, close to the radial bone.

CV 6: 1.5 cun inferior to the center of the umbilicus.

GGV16: 1 cun directly above midpoint of posterior hairline directly below external occipital protuberance in depression between trapezius of both sides.

K 1: Between the ball of the big toe and second toe on sole of the foot.

B 60: Behind the external malleolus, in the depression between the tip of the external malleolus and calcaneus tendon

LI 18 bilaterally: On the side of the neck between the sternocleidomastoid and trapezius muscles at the level of the top of the Adam's apple.

LI 4: Fleshy area between thumb and first finger, near the first metacarpal.

S 36: In the depression on the lateral side of the top of the tibia.

SI 8 bilaterally: On the medial aspect of the elbow, in the depression between the olecranon of the ulna and the medial epicondyle of the humerus.

K 3: In the depression between the medial malleolus and the Achilles tendon, level with the tip of the medial malleolus.

MH 6: On the palmar aspect of the forearm, 2 cun above the transverse crease of the wrist.

TH 5: 2 cun proximal to the dorsal wrist crease between the radius and ulna, close to the radial bone.

SP4: In the depression below the joint at the proximal part of the first metatarsal bone.

SheLi TENS for improving fertility: Apply electrodes to the Chong Mo "sea of blood" acupuncture points SP4, K3, CV2, MH6.

For optimizing endocrine glands, apply TENS electrodes as follows:
Pituitary: LR 14, GB 20.
Adrenals: B 22, CV 6.
Thyroid: ST 9, CV 22, CV 23.

The Shealy-Sorin Gamma PEMF: Every cell in a healthy body has a minus-seventy millivolt charge. When a cell is overstressed, the charge may drop to minus-50. The best way to return cells to their optimal -70 mV charge is the Shealy-Sorin Gamma PEMF. There are other Pulsed Electromagnetic Frequency (PEMF) devices available nationally, but none others put the brain into 40 Hz Gamma, the optimal frequency for brain and body health. This device has been helpful in relieving pain, reducing blood pressure, improving oxygenation, reducing anxiety and depression, and stopping cravings in opioid addicts. More intelligent individuals produce more 40 Hz Gamma activity than people with measurably less intelligence. Application of 40 Hz stimulation the forehead increases the ability to solve complex logical problems, with the benefit being greater in those with lower intelligence.

It can be used for hour or up to 20 hours daily and (as already noted) is safe except for those with an implanted electrical device or in pregnancy.

The Shealy-Sorin Sapphire-Enhanced Scalar: Studies performed at the Shealy-Sorin Wellness Institute demonstrate that exposure to sapphire-enhanced Scalar energy significantly reduces adrenomedullin (ADM), the most important biochemical marker of stress. It also reduces free radicals, inflammation, and blood sugar. In treating Pandas syndrome, it aids in reducing congenital cartilage tumors.

As a marker for impaired hemodynamics, adrenomedullin is the only major ELISA test for your cumulative stress profile; and yet it is not tested at all by clinicians and there is no way to test for it outside of specialized research labs. This seems criminal, since ADM is the single best test for prognosis in cancer patients.

Combining AT and Scalar Healing: As you breathe in, say to yourself "I breathe," and as you breathe out, say "the power of God." As you do so, make it your firm intention to accept and believe that, with each breath, you are focusing the divine power capable of healing every cell in your body. This At exercise can be repeated for any healing and continued for at least twenty minutes.

Crystals: Quartz has been used as a magnifier of healing for thousands of years. In 1988 Shealy found that mentally imprinted quartz crystals led to a 70% long-term improvement in depression, compared with only 28% with glass. Using crushed sapphire worn over the heart, we've found striking reduction in coronary artery calcification in two individuals. More recently, we've run Scalar energy through crushed sapphire, which resulted in overall stress-reduction.

The Shealy-Sorin Wellness Program for Pain & Depression: The alleviation of pain and depression lies at the core of Wellness Institute's healthcare philosophy and mission. Treatment modalities include the following:

Liss CES with Biogenics Neurological Retraining.
SheLi TENS for pain.
Sacred Rings stimulation with SheLi TENS.
Transcutaneous acupuncture.
Gamma PEMF.
Posture pump for spinal problems.
Vibratory music.
Heat therapy.

RelaxMate and light therapy.
HealthRider, vibratory and limbering exercise.
Biogenics Self-Regulation System.
Past-Life Therapy.
Massage.

We invite readers to contact the Wellness Institute and set up a consultation (see Appendix for contact information). Perhaps one or more (or all!) of the abovementioned modalities will prove of benefit.

Pain Lore
(Lore: wisdom, teaching, and knowledge)

Pain is waiting.
Seldom silent. Never asleep.
Always ready to return and remind.
So clever, this pain.

Pain pushes and prods, probes and plays.
Yes, plays.
Plays with us and through us.
She is alluring.
When she arrives we are captivated.
Motivated.
To move and to change.

Pain plays with heads and hearts and limbs.
A maestro conducting a symphony of a soul.

Seductive.
Slow and then building to a crescendo.
Putting us through our paces.
Is that her purpose?

You cannot ignore her. Not any longer.
Melody moves through us.
Rushes, lifts and explodes.
Harmony, then: we grow to live
 with this sound, this hurt.

A prankster now.
We think she is gone but she has changed. A magician.
An ache in the head becomes
Hurt in the heart.

The wand is whisked.
We long to be numbed
With words or whiskey—whatever.
Weary, weakened.

A respite for a while
But *he* returns.
An artist is he—accomplished at that.
Handiwork that leaves us smarting.

A wash in color,
Vibrant blues and purples

Staining us to the quick
With deep, penetrating presence.

A palate of playful perfection is
This pain.
He wants us to move,
Beckons—challenges us to change. And so we do.

Profound, confounding,
Elusive.
In one place and everyplace
Timeless and faceless.
She searches us out to prove her point.

—Georgianne Ginder (September 26, 2002)

CHAPTER FOUR

Forces of the Cosmos at Play: Some Further Avenues to Self-Knowledge

C. Norman Shealy

Here's a question that may have crossed your mind: Does it matter if a reader agrees with all, most, some, or little of the following? (If you agree with none of it, do yourself a favor and stop reading!) I don't expect readers to assent to my every proposition; it's more important that you *understand* the following discussion than that you "buy into" every claim. Throughout this book, my co-authors and I have given science-based evidence for the various complementary/alternative modalities. We know that some will doubt CAM treatments as a matter of course; some people, frankly, are constitutionally incapable of conceiving the "paradigm shifts" underlying holistic practice. Besides, we admit that the various modalities of energy medicine can be theorized in different ways.

Does it *matter* if the chakras are experienced as an energetic reality or are merely "imagined" as an aspect of one's meditation? Does it *matter* if a Reiki master's hands impart real healing energies or have a "placebo effect" upon those who *believe* in the technique? Does it *matter* if prayer reaches to the heavens or remains an "autosuggestion" that becomes self-fulfilling over time? *Does* it matter? Maybe not: "Active imagination" and the "healer effect" and the "placebo effect" and self-hypnosis or "autosuggestion" are themselves well-established modalities of energy medicine. All these proceed from the premise that *the mind leads the body* and, thus, participates in the body's healing.

The topics covered in this chapter are esoteric in a Western sense only; they represent "the wisdom of the ages" as well as "the wisdom of the sages" from Chinese, Hindu-Ayurvedic, and yes, Judeo-Christian mystic tradition. We've been saying all along that health is an expression of body, mind, and spirit. Previous chapters have focused on the body and mind; it's the soul's turn now to receive its due. Actually, that last statement's an oversimplification: Wherever one part goes—body, mind, or spirit—the others follow as a matter of course.

1. Self-Understanding Through the Chakras

Our physical, mental, and emotional conditions are related to the energy centers of our body. Problems with legs relate to our family as well as our community: These belong to the first chakra, the sciatic plexus. Issues of the second chakra—the pelvic plexus—deal with sexuality, finances, and security. The third chakra—the solar plexus—relate to self-esteem and responsibility. The fourth chakra—the energy of the heart—relates to judgment and love. The fifth chakra—centered in the neck—relates to will, to our ability to express our needs and desires. The sixth chakra—situated between and slightly above the eyebrows—relates to our mind and brain, our logic and reason. The seventh chakra—situated at the crown of the head—relates to our connection with soul, spirit, and God. The problems and conditions associated with each chakra follow.

First chakra issues:

Survival, drive, aspiration, and grounding.

Obesity, especially in the legs.

Pain or movement issues with feet and legs.

Sacral pain.

Issues with legs and feet.

Rectal, hemorrhoids, and lower colon problems.

Varicose veins.

Constipation and/or diarrhea.

Anemia, leukemia.

Immune problems.

Second chakra issues:

Sexuality, finances, security.

Menstrual problems or those of ovaries, uterus.

Prostate or testicular problems.

Fertility or reproductive problems.

Bladder problems.

Libido problems.

Hip problems.

Low back pain.

Third chakra issues:

Responsibility and self-esteem.

Stomach and digestive problems.

Disorders of the spleen or lymph system.

Appendicitis.

Liver problems.

Hepatitis.

Pancreas problems.

Diabetes.

Obesity.

Hypoglycemia.

Kidney problems.

Issues with hips or thighs.

Eating and digestive problems.

Colitis.

Gall bladder stones.

Cholecystitis.

Coeliac disease.

Colon cancer.

Fourth chakra issues:

Love and justice.

All varieties of heart disease.

Circulation problems.

Hypertension, also hypotension.

COPD.

Pneumonia, bronchitis.

Lung cancer.

Atrial fibrillation.

Serious immune problems.

Breast cancer and other breast problems.

Chest and thoracic pain.

Asthma.

Scoliosis.

Fifth chakra issues:

Expression of needs and desires.

All problems involving arms and hands.

Thyroid function-under or overactive.

Neck and jaw problems.

Tonsillitis, sore throat, laryngitis.

Lymph gland problems.

Tinnitus, hearing problems, ear infections.

Issues related to nose.

Cervical spine and spinal cord problems.

Sixth chakra issues:

Mental problems, thinking, intuition, creativity.

Eye, vision problems.

Sinus problems.

Headaches, including migraine.

Stroke.

Learning disabilities.

Personality problems.

Seizures.

Memory Issues.

Insomnia and other sleep problems.

Brain tumors.

Depression and anxiety.

Dizziness, vertigo.

Balance problems.

Alzheimer's.

Panic disorder.

Parkinsonism.

Unexplained fatigue.

Dyslexia.

ADHD.

Schizophrenia.

Multiple Sclerosis.

Amyotrophic Lateral Sclerosis.

Nose and sinus-related issues.

Severe ear related issues; deafness.

Learning disabilities or issues related to cognition.

Spinal cord dysfunctions and or nerve related issues.
Depression and anxiety; panic disorders.

Healing adjuncts include crystals, colors, sounds, foods, HERBS AND spices, and behaviors associated with (and supportive of) the health of each specific chakra. Eastern literature on these topics is massive; the following is a mere scratch on the surface but suggestive, nonetheless, of holistic health connections.

First Chakra: Safety.
Color: Red.

Crystal: Ruby.

Forgive all family, community issues and release them to God.

Sound: Note C.

Foods: Red or dark brown foods or drinks, root vegetables such as carrots, sweet potatoes, tomatoes, turnips, radishes, beets, onion, garlic, eggs, meats, beans, tofu, soy. Seeds and nuts: almonds, peanuts.

Herbs and spices: Burdock, cayenne, chive, cloves, clover, dandelion, horse radish, paprika, pepper.

Second Chakra: Security, finances, sexuality.
Color: Orange.

Crystals: Citrine, topaz.

Resolve all issues related to security, finances, sexuality.

Sound: Note D.

Foods: Oranges, high water foods, fats and oils, especially fish, coconut, melons, mangos, strawberries, passion fruit, tangerines, coconut, honey. Seeds and nuts: Pumpkin, almonds, cashews, sunflower and pumpkin seeds, pistachios, walnuts.

Herbs and spices: Anise, celery, cinnamon, cumin, fennel, fenugreek ginger, lily of the valley, marshmallow, melissa, mints, turmeric, cumin, fennel.

Third Chakra: Self-respect, responsibility.

Color: Yellow.

Crystal: Amber.

Resolve all issues related to self-esteem and responsibility.

Sound: Note E.

Foods: Yellow or gold foods: chia, corn, flax, legumes, millet, grains except wheat, corn, gluten free pasta and bread, milk, oatmeal, cheese, yogurt.

Herbs and spices: Anise, cabbage, celery, Chinese cabbage, cinnamon, cilantro, cumin, fennel, ginger, lily of the valley, marshmallow, melissa, mints, turmeric, cumin, fennel.

Fourth Chakra: Love, judgment.

Color: Emerald green.

Crystal: Emerald.

Resolve all issues related to love and justice and fairness.

Sound: Note F.

Foods: Broccoli, chard, celery, collards, dill, green peppers, kale, lettuce, moringa, okra.

Herbs and spices: Basil, cayenne, cilantro; hawthorn berries, jasmine, lavender, marjoram, parsley, rose, sage, thyme, cilantro, parsley, spirulina.

Fifth Chakra: Will, expression of needs and desires.

Color: Deep blue.

Crystal: Blue sapphire.

Resolve all issues related to personal will, needs, desires.

Sound: Note G.

Foods: Blueberries, blue grapes, blue corn and cornmeal, blue potato, blue cheese.

Herbs and spices: Blue crocus, bunga terang.

Sixth Chakra: Reason, logic.

Color: Indigo, blue-purple.

Crystal: Indigo sapphire.

Resolve all issues related to mood.

Sound: Note A.

Foods: Black beans, black cherries, black currants, black olives, black raspberry, black soybeans, blackberry, boysenberries, plums, elderberries, prunes, raisins.

Herbs and spices: Eyebright, juniper, mugwort, poppy, rosemary, lavender, poppyseed.

Seventh Chakra: Spirituality, connection with divine.

Color: Violet purple.

Crystal: Amethyst.

Resolve all spiritual issues.

Sound: Note B.

Foods: Eggplant, passionfruit, purple grapes, *all blessed foods!*

Herbs and spices: Gotu kola, lavender, lotus.

While the energy centers of the chakras are aligned along the spine, they direct and channel *qi* energy through the body's meridian pathways. Eastern acupuncturists have mapped the meridians in precise, minute detail, establishing each meridian point's placement and biological function. What we need to emphasize is the interconnectedness of the chakras and meridians: Taken together, they form a vast energetic highway within the human microcosm.[1]

In *Reading the Body*, Wataru Ohashi describes the holistic foundations of Eastern medicine: The human creature being a unity of body, mind, and spirit, the "Oriental diagnostician views all three realms as one" (p. 10).[2] Within this body-mind-spirit "unity," the whole is greater than the sum of its parts—and that, as we've noted,

---

1 In fact, the flow of energy reaches beyond the material bodies into our surrounding auric fields. Were there world enough and time, I'd write of these, as well.

2 Wataru Ohashi, *Reading the Body* (New York: Penguin, 1991).

is a reigning assumption of holistic medicine generally. Ohashi continues:

> Within the body, each organ is seen in relation to all the others. The health of an individual organ—the liver, for example—depends on the healthy functioning of every other organ.... The liver, heart, spleen, large intestine, and kidneys—to name just a few—are all working in harmony, each one dependent on the others for health. If there is an adequate flow of ki throughout the body, every cell will be nourished with life-giving energy. Every organ will be able to perform its tasks optimally. If the energy is blocked, cells and organs suffocate from lack of ki. (p. 11)

The Japanese "ki" is one of several variants of the universal life-force, *qi*. In Western Tradition, as Ohashi notes, "if we speak of 'the liver' or 'problems of the liver' we are speaking only of physical problems of the organ itself," whereas in Eastern tradition "we could be speaking of the organ itself or of the energy meridian that relates to that organ, and problems affecting that organ or meridian are sometimes physical and sometimes psychological" (p. 12). It is misleading, thus, "to speak of the body as separate from the life energy, or spirit," since the body "is the outward manifestation of [the] spirit."[3]

---

3 Given this body-mind-spirit unity, "every human characteristic—whether emotional, intellectual, or spiritual—has a corresponding physical organ" (Ohashi, p. 12):

> In Oriental diagnosis, we say that the health of the body is directly related to the health of the mind and to personal psychology. We even say that each emotion is associated with a particular organ

Having been blessed by strong powers of intuition (and an equally strong connection to my personal spirit-guide), I have synthesized components of Eastern meridian therapy with Western homeopathy and energy medicine, thus creating a new healing modality—"The Five Sacred Rings," as I've called it. The Sacred Rings are truly revolutionary in their healing potential, serving to wed "the wisdom of the s/ages" with 21st century bioenergetics. Having discussed the Sacred Rings in detail elsewhere,[4] I present a simplified outline of the protocol, below.

2. The Five Sacred Rings

Over the past twenty years, we have discovered in the human body five circuits, which activate specific chemical pathways. These circuits can be stimulated by means of the Shealy GigaTENS unit—a powerhouse of TENS technology capable of frequencies ranging from 52 to 78 billion pulses per second. This latter frequency has been shown by Ukrainian physicists to equal the frequency of

---

or group of organs.... The liver, for example, is related to anger. When the liver is troubled or injured, you have more anger in your life. The kidneys are the seat of the will and control fear. The more troubled the kidneys, the more fear you experience. (Ohashi, p. 12)

The Eastern practitioner, thus, would not "think of taking out a gall bladder or spleen without recognizing that the whole person will be changed, will cease to be who he or she was" (Ohashi, pp. 12-13).

4   For a fuller discussion of the Sacred Rings and Bliss oils, see my book, *Living Bliss: Major Discoveries Along the Holistic Path* (Carlsbad, CA: Hay House, 2014). See also Shealy, *Conversations with G: A Physicians's Encounter with Heaven* (Bloomington, IN: Balboa Press, 2018).

human DNA. Regular SheLi TENS and AlphaStim units do not substantially raise levels of DHEA. The stimulation required can be achieved by application of the GigaTENS—a complex (and pricey) piece of technology—or by application of the five Shealy Bliss oils, each one designed to activate a specific ring. The five circuits or Sacred Rings are as follows:

FIRE: Diseases of Fire include depression, inflammation, hypertension, migraine, diabetes, pain. Stimulation of Fire increases DHEA, the adrenal hormone that is low or deficient in most individuals due to excess stress. In addition to raising DHEA, stimulation of FIRE has been clinically successful in 70 to 80% of patients who have rheumatoid arthritis, migraine, depression, or diabetic neuropathy. Stimulation must be done daily for three months and then at least three times a week to maintain the improvement. Meridian points (for application) are K 3; CV 2, 6, and 18; B 22; MH6; LI 18; GV 20 (behind the ankle bones, on the inside where the ankles touch when standing).

CONCEPTION VESSEL 6: About 1/2 inch below the umbilicus (belly button).

CONCEPTION VESSEL 18: About two inches down from the top of the breastbone.

BLADDER 22: Directly behind the belly button, one inch to either side of the spine.

MASTER OF HEART 6: On the wrists, about one inch up from the palms.

LARGE INTESTINE 18: On the sides of the neck about 1

inch down from the mastoid bones.

GOVERNING VESSEL 20: Top center of the skull, above.

WATER: Diseases of Water include congestion, congestive heart failure, diabetes insipidus, swelling and lymphedema, obesity, and erratic emotions. Stimulation optimizes aldosterone, the hormone responsible for regulation of water and potassium. Theoretically it may help balance emotions. Stimulation of WATER and FIRE together has been found to help significantly in weight loss. The meridian points are SP 4; GV 8, 20; CV 14; B 10, 13; H 7; TH 16.

SPLEEN 4: Run your fingers back along the long bones of the big toe, until you reach a joint on the inside of the foot. Wiggle your toes and you will know you are on the joint.

CONCEPTION VESSEL 14: In the center of your abdomen just below the breastbone.

GOVERNING VESSEL 7.5: Directly behind CV 14 in the center over the spine.

BLADDER 13: Lay your hands over the tops of your shoulders. The tips of your fingers, placed just to the sides of the spine, will now be on B 13.

HEART 7: Feel the space between two tendons on the outer wrists, just beyond the palm; touch the long bone of the small finger.

BLADDER 10: Put your middle fingers one-half inch to both sides of the center of the spine, an inch below the skull.

TRIPLE HEATER 16: Turn your head to the left side and feel the back of the sternocleidomastoid muscle that becomes tight in your right neck; massage the back of that muscle just below the mandible (lower jaw). Then turn your head to the right and do the same thing on the similar area in your left neck.

AIR: Diseases of Air include hearing problems, tinnitus, lung diseases such as asthma, COPD, emphysema, autism, Down's Syndrome, Fainting, and mental problems. Stimulation raises neurotensin, a neurochemical which helps fat metabolism but is also a neuroleptic. More importantly, AIR raises oxytocin, the nurturing hormone. Treatment is excellent for depression and anxiety. Autism can be treated by a combination of AIR and EARTH: This combination appears to assist in establishing a meditative state or "simultaneity of thought." Meridian points are Sp 1a; LIV 3; S 36, 9; B 60; LI 16; GV 20.

EARTH: Diseases of Earth are chronic fatigue, fibromyalgia, paralysis, osteoporosis, stroke, ALS, Parkinsonism, immune problems, pain, kidney and liver disease, addiction. which raises calcitonin significantly. Stimulation raises calcitonin, a hormone produced in the thyroid and the key regulator of calcium metabolism in bone. Calcitonin is a powerful tool for maintaining strong bones. Calcitonin is also 40 to 60 times as strong as morphine in reducing pain. Stimulation of this ring may help addiction, ground the personality, and serve as an adjunct in rebuilding the body. Some individuals need

EARTH and FIRE (along with Iodoral supplements) to restore thyroid function. Meridian points are K 1; B 60, 54; LI 16; S 9; SI 17; GV 20.

CRYSTAL: Diseases of Crystal are degenerative diseases, wear and tear, and co-factor with diseases of Earth. Within seven days of regular use, stimulation reduces free radicals significantly. Free radicals are the destructive chemical toxins that invade the body by what we eat, drink, breathe in, and absorb through our skin, damaging cells and causing premature aging. Theoretically, reducing free radicals could be the single most important adjunct for enhancing health and longevity. Meridian points are SP 4; G 11, 30.5; CV 8.5, 14.5, 23; GV 4.5, 7.5, 14.5, 20.

The Methuselah Promise: Healthy "youthing." In addition to the Ring of Fire, stimulation of the Rings of Crystal and Earth should optimize overall health and longevity. Start using the specific elemental Bliss oils. Earth increases calcitonin, great for bone strength and general well-being. Crystal markedly reduces Free Radicals, the cause of disease, aging and death! These and/or the RejuvaMatrix may well be all that is needed.

There are three proven ways to regenerate your telomeres. Telomeres are the tips of your DNA and shrink 1% every year, if you have good health habits. You can regenerate them 3.5% every year, potentially prolonging *healthy* life to 120 years and beyond, using the following:

- SheLI TENS stimulation daily of the Rings of Fire, Earth and Crystal.
- Use daily Fire, Earth and Crystal Bliss.
- Use the Rejuvamatrix mattress (with embedded Tesla coil) one hour each night.

And then there's the "youth" hormone ...

EPITALON: The so-called "youth" hormone, epitalon is the hormone of the pineal gland, ultimately the master control hormone for the pituitary and general homeostasis (especially of the immune system). It is the only known hormone to increase lifespan significantly in humans! It is available at the Shealy-Sorin Wellness Institute to be taken subcutaneously once a month or a triple dose every three months. You might want to have tested your telomeres and DHEA before starting, to monitor your progress! This can be done at first visit.

From the microcosm of the human body and its meridians, we move on to the macrocosm and its influences upon body, mind, and soul.

3. Astrology and Personality

In addition to the workings of the chakras, I sense in every individual the influence of their basic astrological pattern. If I were to write, "this person is energetic, optimistic, and enthusiastic," it might sound like I was describing qualities associated with extraversion. If I were to write that another person was "friendly but independent and occasionally detached," it might sound like I was applying criteria of openness. But I'd not be drawing from the Five-Factor Model as described in Chapter 2; instead, I'd be drawing from the wisdom of astrology. For instance, when I know the sun, moon, north node, and rising sign of an individual, I gain insights into her personality that no trait model—not the MBTI or "the Big Five" or any other model of personality testing—can supply. Of course, I still have to learn who that person is individually. In addition, the character of both parents influences everything about that person, even beyond astrological influences. And, as one very wise intuitive said, in that unknown DNA is stored all the genetic information of our ancestors.

It should not come as a surprise that the ancients, in their wisdom, had their own instruments of categorizing and predicting personality types. Whereas the Five-

Factor model is a few decades old, astrology extends back for millennia and was implicated in European medicine well into the seventeenth century. I would add that the development of astronomy as "science" came at a high spiritual price. With the observations of Copernicus, Kepler, and other early astronomers, the motion of the planets through the solar system was more accurately measured and predicted; but the *resonances* of those planets and their influences upon human life and history was suppressed—though never entirely forgotten.[5]

SUN SIGNS refer to the Sun's position in the zodiac at the time of one's birth. The zodiac consists of twelve sun signs, which are further divided into four groups of three, each group reflecting one of the four classical elements

---

5   Let's make this explanation simple: The cosmos consists of energies, and energies interact. The planets resonate their influences outward, and, at the time of one's birth, the strongest planetary and astrological influences leave their imprint upon people "born under their sign."

People who have not developed their powers of intuition and sensitivity might say, "I don't feel the effects of Mars or Libra or any of that cosmic stuff." But have you considered the fact that the earth rotates at dizzying speed—1,000 miles per hour at the equator—and is hurtling through space, circling the sun at 67,000 miles per hour? *And do you feel it?* Here's a cosmic irony: There are 326,000,000,000,000,000,000 *gallons* (that's 326 million trillion *gallons*) of water in the ocean and, every day, the moon's gravitational pull lifts these trillions of gallons upwards—as little as three feet on some coastlines, as much as fifty feet on others. The seawater responds to the moon's pull, *but we don't.* We don't even "feel" it.

By the way, the great Galileo Galilei (1564-1642), discoverer of the moons of Jupiter and Saturn's rings, was officially a professor of medical astrology at the University of Padua. In the 17ᵗʰ century, it was believed that certain medical procedures would "take" only with the assistance of planetary influences: Back then, a physician studied both *what to do* and *when to do it* (when, say, to apply a poultice or an emetic or to bleed a patient), all in accordance with celestial influences upon specific organs of the body. In fact, some two dozen of Galileo's astrological charts survive, made to determine the opportune time to begin a patient's medical treatment.

of Fire (hot and dry), Earth (cold and dry), Air (hot and moist), and Water (cold and moist). (Isn't it brilliant how the macrocosm and microcosm mirror each other? The Sacred Rings were not named randomly, after all.)

FIRE SIGNS: Aries, Leo and Sagittarius are energetic, optimistic and enthusiastic.

EARTH SIGNS: Taurus, Capricorn and Virgo are secure, serious and practical.

AIR SIGNS: Gemini, Libra and Aquarius are sociable, friendly, independent, more detached but good communicators.

WATER SIGNS: Pisces, Scorpio and Cancer (moonchild) are emotional, intuitive, and feeling.

A more detailed description of each sign and its dominant traits follows.

ARIES: The Warrior, is absorbed with self-interests, fearless, often successful, very direct, honest, occasionally rash, forcefully optimistic, highly energetic.

TAURUS: The Builder, is tranquil, likes to be alone, lover of home, strong and healthy in constitution, artistic and art-loving, very self-controlled.

GEMINI: The Communicator, is sign of the twins, versatile, a fast thinker who can change course suddenly, dislikes being pinned down, is charming, persuasive, Mercurial.

CANCER (MOONCHILD): The Preserver, is the most emotionally up-or-down of all signs, generous, a lover of food with a green thumb, can be lonely or shy, caring, gentle.

LEO: The Leader of the world, is commanding, stately, a great teacher or politician, is regal, forgiving and sympathetic, loyal, generous, affectionate, but makes a power enemy.

VIRGO: The Perfectionist, is dependable, secure, gentle, somewhat restless, prudent, as critical of self as of anything, is prudent, organized, more sure of self than any other; the most conscientious.

LIBRA: The Socializer, is romantic but fickle, demands justice and fairness, likes order and harmony.

SCORPIO: The Transformer, is intelligent and the most manipulating, over-sexed and the most passionate.

SAGITTARIUS: The Explorer, is the-foot-in-mouth blunt, restless, honest, lovable, intelligent, high-spirited, spiritual, prone to accidents, clownish.

CAPRICORN: The Pragmatist, is businesslike, creative, conscientious, organized, determined, dependable.

AQUARIUS: The Inventor, is a butterfly chasing a rainbow, imprecise and curiously experimental, freedom-loving, lives in the future, a lover of the unknown and mystical.

PISCES: The Dreamer, is creative, artistic, tolerant, free of greed, rose-colored, can swim to the top or to the bottom, represents death and serenity, is a master of satire.

INFLUENCE OF THE MOON: The moon influences mood, femininity, love, and emotions, so when the moon is in one of the astrological signs, that sun sign influences the moon's effects. The sun represents action and the moon represents reaction in emotions. During a new moon, thinking becomes much more irrational. A most satisfying relationship occurs when one's moon is in the sun sign of another person. The full moon increases libido and erratic behavior. The most remarkable effect of the moon is on plants: Never plant in an unfavorable time! (On this point of practical wisdom, see *Farmer's Almanac Gardening Calendar.*)

NORTH NODE: The north node represents one's greatest challenges in this life, while the south node represents one's greatest karmic strength.

RISING SIGN: This determines the ways that you wish to present yourself to the world. The time of your birth is another strong influence upon your personality.

BORN BETWEEN MIDNIGHT AND 2 A.M.
You make wise use of money, are persuasive and family-oriented.

BORN BETWEEN 2 A.M. AND 4 A.M.
You believe in yourself, dislike being alone, and make friends easily.

BORN BETWEEN 4 A.M. AND 6 A.M.
You're a "hopeless romantic" and attract friends easily.

BORN BETWEEN 6 A.M. AND 8 A.M.
A perfectionist, you love meditation and enjoy time alone.

BORN BETWEEN 8 A.M. AND 10 A.M.
You are shy but can grow into being the center of attention.

BORN BETWEEN 10 A.M. AND NOON
You are ambitious and driven to succeed.

BORN BETWEEN NOON AND 2 P.M.
You like being active and make a great student as well as a great teacher.

BORN BETWEEN 2 P.M. AND 4 P.M.
You're lucky and often take advantage of that luck.

BORN BETWEEN 4 P.M. AND 6 P.M.
You're an optimist who overcome obstacles easily; you enjoy relationships and are kind.

BORN BETWEEN 6 P.M. AND 8 P.M.
A hard worker, you sometimes push yourself too hard; you're bright and understand others well.

BORN BETWEEN 8 P.M. AND 10 P.M.
You are generous and giving.

BORN BETWEEN 10 P.M. AND MIDNIGHT
You're a born leader with good judgment.

Now, while the astrological influences are significant, you can override them or embellish them with your personal drive. If you have trouble doing your own astrological interpretation, consult a good astrologer.

Karma: Past-life involvement in present-day life problems.

Life is an opportunity to explore innumerable pathways, to clean up old karma, and to understand yourself. Self-understanding starts, perhaps paradoxically, with understanding your parents: who they are, what they mean, and why you were given to each other—for the choice of parents is the first great meaningful act of one's present life. At a soul level, before we incarnate, we meet with our angelic guides and are told we need to develop one or more personality traits— security, say, or flexibility, or forgiveness. Sometimes we are given more than one choice of parents; sometimes, seemingly, the Universe chooses for us. I will never be able in this life to understand why we might wind up with crazy, mean, unloving or otherwise harmful parents; but, considering what has presented itself in the 32,000 plus patients I've seen over the years, I've learned that anything is possible.

I have often said, "I did not have the courage to choose abusive parents." I had the most nurturing parents I can imagine, and I am forever grateful for this experience. On the other hand, I have encountered outside my family more than one psychopath, which I can only accept as karma. While many fundamentalist Christians refuse to accept the reality of reincarnation, I have recalled at least thirty of my previous lives, in several of which I was not my current benevolent self. And, having guided hundreds of individuals to find meaning in unfinished anger, guilt, depression or anxiety carried over from a previous life, I can state that I do not "believe in" reincarnation; rather, *I know it* as a fundamental fact of the universe. It's the sort of knowledge that defines reality for me, providing a framework for my understanding of the world, myself, and others.

Our souls have been around for many eons and we have had many experiences—good, bad, and in between. (And between-life experiences can also be valuable, too!) In conducting hundreds of guided past-life regressions, I've come to conclude that most current life problems, both physical and mental, contain some unfinished anger, guilt, depression, or trauma left over from a previous life. [6]

---

6   If you cannot visit a good past-life therapist locally, the best past-life intuitive that I know is Kevin Ryerson, whom you can find on the internet.

4. An Art of Loving

> True love is like ghosts, which everybody talks
> about and few have seen.
>
> **—François de La Rochefoucauld**

La Rochefoucauld (1618-1680) is right: We talk about love all the time, as if experts in the art of loving. And most of us have "felt" its unearthly presence, though we haven't in fact "seen" it—that is, *known it*, experiencing it fully, consciously, conscientiously. Until we can say what it is, how can we claim to possess it, much less to practice it? In our hunt for definitions, I begin with *The Book of Urantia*, which declares that "love is the desire to do good to others."[7] I'm especially fond of this definition, as it points to the main purpose in life itself. A true understanding of the interconnectedness of everything (and an appreciation for the remarkable physical power and beauty of the universe) encourages us to do good in life. Love is for giving, not taking; it's for support, compassion, tolerance, charity, hope, faith, joy, forgiveness, and serenity. Its opposites are judgmentalism, guilt, fear, an unwillingness to let go, anxiety, anger, frustration, resentment. To do good is commonsensical: It's the Golden Rule in action.

---

[7] *Urantia Book*, "Characteristic Manifestations of Love" (648.3), Urantia Foundation (https://www.urantia.org), accessed 28 March 2020.

One's ability to feel, give, and receive love is based largely on the nurturing one received from conception through at least the first seven years of life. Most stress-related diseases have their origins in a child's perceived abandonment, lack of love, or actual harm—an emotional or physical (including sexual) abuse. In articulating a "hierarchy of needs," Abraham Maslow (1908-1970) outlined a model of human development that begins with physical survival and culminates in spiritual transcendence.[8] We all need air, water, food, clothing, and shelter: These are the basics, essential for survival. But we need more. We need nurturance—a love that provides emotional security, models friendship and intimacy, and fosters self-esteem. Sometimes, the lack of parental nurturing leads to lifelong depression, which Eysenck (as we've noted) found to be a major cause of death from cancer. And parental abuse leads to lifelong anger, the number one cause of death by heart attack. Childhood/adolescent psychology teaches us that successful nurturing aids in developing an autonomous personality. As we noted in our discussion of Five-Factor trait theory, an autonomous, self-actualized individual can expect to live thirty-four years longer on average than an individual whose life lacked nurturing.

Self-actualized individuals recognize that unhappiness is a result of unfulfilled, unrealized desires. They learn to

---

8 See his *Religions, Values, and Peak Experiences* (Columbus, OH: Ohio State University Press, 1964). In fact, the traits associated with self-actualization largely mirror the FFT personality trait of conscientiousness.

divorce with joy the situations that cause anger, anxiety, resentment, depression. This liberation from anger leads to the transcendent will of the soul, which allows us to accept "with serenity the things that cannot be changed."[9] It frees us from judgment and need to know why.

For centuries poets, philosophers, and theologians have expounded upon the concept of love. This chapter takes an eclectic approach, asking readers to explore their own beliefs in relation to other people's thoughts and writings. The most important questions you can ask relate to love, for love is the ultimate life path. As you read, pause after any question or intriguing statement: Close your eyes and *feel* your response. No one can answer these questions for

---

9 This is the famous serenity prayer of American theologian, Reinhold Niebuhr (1892-1971). Most people know it in part, though not in full (http://skdesigns.com/internet/articles/prose/niebuhr/serenity_prayer):

God, give us grace to accept with serenity
the things that cannot be changed,
Courage to change the things
which should be changed,
and the Wisdom to distinguish
the one from the other.

Living one day at a time,
Enjoying one moment at a time,
Accepting hardship as a pathway to peace,
Taking, as Jesus did,
This sinful world as it is,
Not as I would have it,
Trusting that You will make all things right,
If I surrender to Your will,
So that I may be reasonably happy in this life,
And supremely happy with You forever in the next.
Amen.

you. No one possesses your own final truth except you. So, please take time to complete the following Love Attitude Inventory. (As always in this book, you should write out your answers.)

What is Love?

We're told, "love thy neighbor as thyself" (Mark 12.31). *How* does one love one's neighbor as one's self?

"And God so loved the world that he gave his only begotten son that, whosoever shall believe in him, shall not perish but have everlasting life" (John 3.16). *What does it mean to you, personally?*

Is love stronger than like?

or

Is like greater than love?

Is love an attitude or an activity?

Is love an emotional response, the fulfilling of a desire?

Is love a spiritual act?

Is sex a spiritual act?

What is unconditional love?

If there is such a thing as unconditional love, is there unconditional sex?

Does unconditional love require practice?

Does the commitment to love unconditionally attract people to us who are *difficult* to love?

Are we selective in showing love, or can we love without judgment, without prejudice?

Is it possible to love one's enemies? To love criminals and murderers?

Is there more to the Golden Rule than altruism?

Common dictionaries vary little in their definitions of love and they often neglect such concepts as unconditional love, spiritual love, and love as extolled in the Bible. Here's *Funk and Wagnall's Standard Dictionary of the English Language* (1958):

> love (1uv) n. A strong, complex emotion or feeling causing one to appreciate, delight in and crave the presence or possession of another and to please or promote the welfare of the other; devoted affection or attachment.
>
> Specifically, such feeling between husband and wife or lover and sweetheart.
>
> One who is beloved; a sweetheart.
>
> Sexual passion, or the gratification of it.
>
> A very great interest or fondness.
>
> In tennis, a score of nothing. [Now *that's* a fascinating meaning!]

As my friend Dr. Robert Leichtman wrote to me some years ago, "It always amazes me that love is usually defined as a noun—a static state of being such and such." Leichtman's letter continues:

But the dynamism of love is missed unless we discuss it as a verb rather than a noun. While we can know love and be loved, it is far more important to us and the world we live in to love others by being helpful and kind to them. Love is also a motive. Sometimes, the experience of love is only a state of pleasant sentiment—useless to all but that person. But when love impels us to be supportive, caring, rescuing, and redeeming, then it comes alive in us, driving us to bring new healing energy into the world. Unless the love we experience penetrates to the heart of our values and motivates us to express it as acts of goodwill, then it is as dead as the faith that is felt but not accompanied by the works which would demonstrate it.[10]

Amen, I say.

So, let's consider what else the dictionary leaves out. We'll start with soul-love, which is the yearning or outgoing of the soul toward something regarded as excellent, beautiful, or desirable. Love, in this sense, denotes something spiritual and reciprocal, such as can have no place in connection with worldly objects that minister to the senses.

***Philia* or "brotherly love"** is a love between equals, serving no other purpose than to further that other person's life. Though other expressions of love may be more intimate, intense, or passionate, we suspect that *philia* is a necessary ingredient—perhaps a precondition, even a foundation—

---

10 Letter from Robert R. Leichtman, M.D., October 21, 1989. Author's personal correspondence.

of them all. The love of friendship should begin early in childhood. The feeling of bonding with individuals of similar interests has an almost unlimited variety: Of love's many expressions, friendship is most various of all, in that it binds individuals, families, organizations, communities, states, countries together.

It is largely through friendships that we learn tolerance and acceptance. No one is perfect. When we like someone, we tend to look beyond their imperfections, treating their idiosyncratic behaviors as eccentricities rather than as great flaws. And even though some friends grow apart as we move on, there are a few who remain throughout most of one's life. "Greater love hath no man than this, that a man lay down his life for his friends" (John 15.13): In its highest sense, the *philia* that kindles one's lifelong commitment to a spouse is the greatest human equivalent of divine love. In the ideal marriage bonding, the only thing that comes close is the love of parents for their children.

Self-Love is typically misunderstood as selfishness, whereas selfishness is caused by a *lack* of self-love. Scripture tells us to "love thy neighbour as thyself" (Matthew 22.39). If it's a virtue to love one's neighbor, then surely it's a virtue to love oneself. If you want, call it *caring* for the self: Call it self-respect, self-understanding, self-acceptance, and a desire to do good to/for oneself. It won't surprise that people who are self-actualized and conscientious practice self-care, and that people with low self-esteem are lacking in self-love. (Do you see, then, why self-love is an important ingredient in health?) Selfishness and self-love are actually opposites. In sum: you cannot truly love others unless you learn first to love yourself.

Love of God is as powerful an experience as any available to humankind, in that it leads to transcendance—a dissolution of ego-boundaries that merges the self with/in the divine. Properly understood, the experience of divine love is to the soul what erotic love (again, properly understood) is to the body: In merging with another being, we become larger than ourselves and "lose ourselves" (albeit temporariliy) in the experience. Mystic unions of this sort allow us to become one with the universe. Though mystic union is rare and fleeting, it takes only one such experience—one instance of the enveloping divine presence—to convince us from that moment on that God is good, that the universe is kind, and that "all shall be well, and all shall be well, and all manner of thing shall be well," as the great English mystic, Julian of Norwich (1342-*ca.* 1416), declares in her spiritual autobiography, *Revelations of Divine Love.*

In discussing divine love, I prefer the insights of mystics over the orthodoxies of theologians. The masculinist pronoun that names God "our father" should not prevent us from experiencing the maternal nurterance of unconditional divine love. When God "became" man or was "made" male, the Judeo-Christian God-image became masculinist in demanding obedience and doling out punishments and rewards. Historically, patriarchal culture tends to stereotype a father's love as conditional—as purchased by loyalty and obedience—and, for that reason, as a love easily lost. In contrast, a mother's love remains unconditional. The patriarchal God of Luther and Calvin was an angry God, strict in "his" punishments and irresistible in "his" power. A real mother will love you even when you sin. In his declaration of God as "the absolute nothing," Meister Eckhart (*ca.* 1260- *ca.* 1328) revels in paradox: There's no question in Eckhart's mind *that* "God is." But our human powers of perception cannot say *what* "God is." Our experience of the divine exceeds language. Certainly God is neither male nor female. The categories of being within the material world are too small a container. The divine essence remains a mystery, though God's goodness can be glimpsed in nature.

We stand in awe of this universe: What is revealed to the naked eye is awesome, what telescopes and space instruments show even more so. The least inspiration from this magnificent creation must lead one to want to know its creator. If the material universe—the macrocosm—is awesome, how much greater is the microcosm—our own substance and being. The human body is a magnificent creation, the mind greater still, the soul greatest of all. Thinking sets in motion a certainty of spiritual forces. The universal awareness that there is a power greater than all human beings has led to a wide variety of God-images and theologies (literally, "ways of talking about God"). There is equally compelling awareness that "human *being*" is a temporary state and that our consciousness continues beyond bodily death. Eons of reports of near-death experience and thousands of reports of proven memories of previous lives convince us that the soul continues. Despite cultural and religious rivalries, we see many similarities in Judaism, Christianity, Sufi Islam, Buddhism, and Hinduism. These and other religions awaken our "God consciousness" and sooth our fears of death.

Saint Francis of Assisi (1181-1226), the patron saint of animals and famous for his reverence for all creation, composed his "Canticle of Brother Sun and Sister Moon" in praise of God's works:[11]

> Praised be my Lord God with all creatures;
> And especially our brother the sun,
> Which brings us the day and the light;
> Fair is he, and shining with a very great splendor:
> O Lord, he signifies you to us!
> Praised be my Lord for our sister the moon,
> And for the stars,
> Which God has set clear and lovely in heaven.
>
> Praised be my Lord for our brother the wind

---

11 I give a modern translation published on the church website, *Caritas* (https://www.caritas.org/2010/04/canticle-of-the-sun-prayer-for-climate-justice). Poignantly, the site calls his canticle "a prayer for climate justice."

And for air and cloud, calms and all weather,
By which you uphold in life all creatures.

Praised be my Lord for our sister water,
Which is very serviceable to us,
And humble, and precious, and clean.

Praised be my Lord for brother fire,
Through which you give us light in the darkness;
And he is bright, and pleasant, and very mighty,
And strong.

Praised be my Lord for our mother the Earth,
Which sustains us and keeps us,
And yields diverse fruits,
And flowers of many colors, and grass.

"Blessed are those who endure in peace," the poem continues, for "By You Most High, they will be crowned." How delightful—and how mysterious—to think of the sun and moon as our brother and sister!

While all of nature—earth, water, air, fire—earns the saint's praise, it's to the sun and its light that St. Francis gives preeminence. Creation began with light—"God said, *let there be light*..."—and the light that illumines the physical world has its analog in spiritual enlightenment, which guides us in truth and gives hope. Meditation and prayer keep us on the spiritual path that leads to enlightenment.

From my work with thousands of individuals suffering from illness, pain, anxiety, and depression, I can say that the greatest spiritual needs appear to be for personal self-esteem, forgiveness, tolerance, and serenity.

Georgianne Ginder on Prayer as Therapy (Prayer-apy):

When people say to me—especially now when I am ill and, as of late, more and more and visibly so—"I will pray for you," what do I think? What do I take away from that? Are they sincere? (Does that really matter?) And just what does that *truly* mean, those five words "I will pray for you"? Will I feel the prayers and will they help me to see, to walk better, to talk, chew, and swallow without pain, to be released from the fears and the weakness? Will I feel less isolated in my world of pain and aloneness ...? How will I know? Or maybe *they* feel better saying that, so that they can be released from any further obligation? Is it my business or theirs?

I have said those words to others and I know that I sometimes forget ... to pray ... and soon even forget about them. I may have become too busy or too preoccupied.

But God does not forget. He heard me say it! So He knows and is right in there, doing the heavy lifting.

Maybe that is it. Maybe all is Well indeed, and so it is that God and I and all of us ... succeed. Indeed!

Those five words said often and often on the run or off the cuff may feel at times like a retort, something that one just says ... like "I appreciate that" or "Have a nice day" or 'My pleasure" or "No prob." (I read a while back that saying *my pleasure* does wonders—even if it is sort of fake—in contrast to *no problem*, which, sadly, often elicits the opposite vibe in our systems. Good to know and now we're good to go, no?! My pleasure and your treasure. *Ah!*)

But the key lies in the response, for in some way you and I *do* respond. As I hurt so with various syndromes (which I try to ignore), what I understand and cannot ignore is that I require genuine and earnest deep-tissue conversation, connection, support, love, presence, and sustenance—not that off the cuff or on the fly stuff. Indeed from the Most High, but too from the most significant of others. But in the last years many of us cannot find the time and place to be available and present. Our significant others—spouses, children, parents, friends, sisters and brothers—are on the go. Still, we spirit/mind/emotional/ physical/social beings require this presiding presence as we require all forms of nutrition. Period. And that's why so many find it hard to heal.

Yet, as I ponder earnestly the power of prayer that is, I grow so deeply aware of and in tune with that someone who is tapping into and harnessing that beloved spiritual force of eternal connection and protection. It's a power of truth, salvation and regeneration, despite the actual and or perceived "physical" manifestation and outcome. The power and the potential of prayer? Healing, lending, sending, and perhaps even that "cure," which can and does stir the soul and all the rest. What exactly is that substance, that resonance, that harmonization? An exquisitely gentle and forceful grace, an energy and power that one can sense, resonate with, feel, inhale, touch and, too, can abide with and dwell within and among. It is the enthusiastic *knowing* and feeling ... which is salvation. (June 7, 2013)

Meeting Your Soulmate: Occasionally you meet one whose soul awakens in you the most intense feelings of physical, mental, emotional, and divine love. In the *Symposium*, Plato writes of love as a "longing for completion." For humans, as Plato's myth-maker Socrates tells us, "were originally created with four arms, four legs and a head with two faces. Fearing their power, Zeus split them into two separate parts, condemning them to spend their lives in search of their other halves." This sense of spiritual incompleteness turns true love into an attraction: for when a person "meets the other half, the actual half of himself,... the pair are lost in an amazement of love and friendship and intimacy and one will not be out of the other's sight, as I may say, even for a moment." I know what Plato's Socrates is talking about!

I have been blessed twice in this lifetime, first and for 53 years in sharing my life with Mary-Charlotte "Chardy" Bayles, with whom I shared three previously known lives of true love. Thanks to Air Bliss and the Liss Cranial Stimulator, I coped for the two years needed to deal with her loss in 2011. Then in June 2015, I met Sergey Sorin, with whom I shared five known previous lives. I "knew" him when I walked into the room where he was teaching Sound Medicine and recognized him as a companion in a previous life, when we were both close to St. Francis. Knowing him now gives me more meaning for life than anyone I have known, much like the meaning of my life with Chardy: *agape* love at its purest.

I cannot overstate the role that soul-love plays in restoring meaning, joy, purpose, and health to people's lives. When love is powerful enough to motivate you to meet your soulmate, a true soul connection, though very rare, becomes very real. And here's what the experience of soul-love teaches:

That true love is finding your soulmate in your best friend; that giving your soul is better than giving your heart or body; that the happiness of the other person becomes more essential than your own; that reality is at last better than your dreams; that you can be fully at ease with and accepting of yourself when you are with your soul-companion. So, if your life is truly blessed, you will meet that person who totally transforms you at all levels of being. Rest assured that some of the people you've met have been with you in a previous life; often, you'll become fast friends in this present life, as well. (Plato's right: The divided soul's longing for completion in love extends across lifetimes.)

Spend some time reflecting on each of the following quotes and what each means to you.

It is not a lack of love, but a lack of friendship that makes unhappy marriages.

—Friedrich Nietzsche

Being deeply loved by someone gives you strength, while loving someone deeply gives you courage.

—Lao Tzu

Love is that condition in which the happiness of another person is essential to your own.

—Robert A. Heinlein, *Stranger in a Strange Land*

Love looks not with the eyes, but with the mind,
And therefore is winged Cupid painted blind.
   —William Shakespeare, *A Midsummer Night's Dream*

Love is like the wind, you can't see it but you can feel it.
   —Nicholas Sparks, *A Walk to Remember*

The best thing to hold onto in life is each other.
   —Audrey Hepburn

"I love you" begins by I, but it ends up by you.
   —Charles de Leusse

Let's end this list with a quote from Dr. Seuss:

I need you like a heart needs a beat.

To Parent or Not to Parent?

Next to the love of one's spouse is, *or should be*, the love of one's children. And yet, in an old newspaper column, Ann Landers wrote that 70% of ten thousand people who wrote to her wished they had never had children! To that sad anecdote, add the fact that 40% of American children are born out of wedlock. Marriage is itself no guarantee of a happy childhood, since 50% of American marriages wind up in divorce court—and parental divorce is one of the greatest traumas a child can endure. Consider, further, that a mere

30% of Americans self-report as happy! Adding up these stats, we calculate that *at least* 70% of American children lack the single most important requirement for emotional health—a sense of being wanted and supported by loving, well-adjusted parents. Speaking of a lack of common sense! It is a serious lack of conscientiousness even to risk having children outside of a well-adjusted marriage. Sex outside marriage is among the many behaviors that can ruin life for both parents and children alike. Condoms, diaphragms, and other methods of birth control are never 100% effective or safe. And, in the long run, birth control pills are among the worst inventions of mainstream medicine, with serious (indeed, life-threatening) complications that can ruin the endocrine system of the woman forever.

Put simply, the decision to parent is life-altering and ought not to be subject to whim chance (e.g., a broken condom). In no area of our lives as social beings is conscientiousness more desperately needed.

Hormonal Nurturing.

Children need remarkable love and nurturing, crucially during the first nine months of life but continuing through birth and the first seven years into adolescence. When a couple consciously decides to have a child and blesses its conception and growth *in utero,* the mother produces daily bursts of oxytocin, the bonding and nurturing hormone. These bursts of oxytocin effectively bond the child naturally with the mother; this maternal bond provides a foundation for future healthy attachments that the child will development throughout life. We've already noted the 40% of America's children born out of wedlock: What of them? Many, unfortunately, look forward to a lifetime of health issues, starting with premature birth, poor weight gain, and respiratory problems. Statistics tell us that they'll face greater challenges in learning, socialization, and self-esteem—to which I'd add an internal spiritual disharmony. Even if the pregnancy is wanted and blessed, that nurturing hormone can be blocked: If the mother is induced into labor, given a spinal anesthetic, or has a Caesarean section, then her normal labor output of massive amounts of oxytocin will be blocked. So, at the crucial moment of birth, the child misses that essential biochemical blessing.

This initial oxytocin loss can be overcome if the parents are truly loving and nurturing. But if some major trauma is experienced during those formative first seven years, a child's normal oxytocin system may be blocked for life. Note that "any kind of abuse, whether ... physical, sexual, emotional, or verbal, can cause trauma" (*Living Bliss* p. 14). But, short of catastrophic accident, violence, or illness, the most traumatic—and common—childhood trauma is parental divorce. Many of our readers are themselves children of divorce and can attest to this life-altering trauma, worse even than the death of a parent.[12]

While not obviously abusive, divorce does interrupt the nurturing process. So, while the children of divorce may not be in physical danger, their sense of loss and insecurity will, like an emotional and psychic wound, carry forward into adulthood.

But, while the wound is registered emotionally and psychologically, it's the hormonal aspect that warrants our attention. Let's by all means keep up the life-coaching and counselling, but let's trade in the antidepressants and anti-anxiety medications for oxytocin. As I write in *Living Bliss*,

There is a huge body of evidence indicating that oxytocin deficiency influences a wide spectrum of disorders, including autism, attention deficit/hyperactivity disorder (ADHD), depression, obsessive-compulsive disorder (OCD), borderline personality, addiction, and schizophrenia. In fact, almost all psychotherapy from the past 200 years has been related to these problems. I feel shock and dismay when I think that therapists have been attempting to change personality within their patients without resetting the thermostat that actually controls it—which is oxytocin! That's why I am suggesting

---

12 Statistics gathered from *The Longevity Project* paint a gloomy picture of parental divorce, whose "long-term health effects ... were often devastating—it was indeed a risky circumstance that changed the pathways of many of the young [Project] participants" (p. 80). As Friedman and Martin note, "children from divorced families died almost five years earlier on average than children from intact families. Parental divorce, not parental death, was the risk. In fact, parental divorce during childhood was the single strongest social predictor of early death, many years into the future" (p. 80).

that a different approach is needed. While I fully accept that nutritional factors, social circumstances, and environmental conditions are all part of the picture of how we turn into functioning adults in our society, I also believe that boosting oxytocin actually has the potential to make a far greater impact and improvement on our lives than just about anything else. (pp. 15-16)

In our life's work as healers, what we find most needed is an attitude of forgiveness—the forgiving of someone from early childhood. No matter what the original damage, it is impossible for an individual to move up the spiritual ladder without forgiving everyone who is felt to have been harmful. This conscious act of forgiveness does not mean accepting or tolerating abuse. But it does require a total emotional detachment and release of the blamed person into the hands of God.

Let me end this chapter with a sonnet by English poet, Elizabeth Barrett Browning (1806 – 1861). This marvelous lyric seems to contain, in miniature, virtually every expression of love described above. It, too, is worth reading in full:

How do I love thee? Let me count the ways.
I love thee to the depth and breadth and height
My soul can reach, when feeling out of sight
For the ends of being and ideal grace.
I love thee to the level of every day's

Most quiet need, by sun and candlelight.
I love thee freely, as men strive for right.
I love thee purely, as they turn from praise.
I love thee with the passion put to use
In my old griefs, and with my childhood's faith.
I love thee with a love I seemed to lose
With my lost saints. I love thee with the breath,
Smiles, tears, of all my life; and, if God choose,
I shall but love thee better after death.

There's soul-love here as well as friendship; there's a childlike feeling of safety-in-dependence as well as the fierce unconditional love of a mother; there's an affirmation of freedom and of responsibility; there's a "passion" that's both erotic—physical—and "pure," reflected in the "quiet need" of daily companionship; and there's recognition that love not only continues, but grows "after death." If we could all love as well as Elizabeth Barrett, we'd be in a better place.

The Coronavirus and Soul Growth: An Epilogue

Among my favorite passages from the *Edgar Cayce Readings* are his discussions of the soul gaining or losing in a given past life and how these may provide challenges— or blessings—in one's present life. The current pandemic provides everyone perhaps their biggest opportunities to gain or lose! I'm also reminded of my concept that religion is the "fight for God," whereas mysticism is the "search for God." At this delicate moment, let's keep up the search. During days and weeks of lockdown, stay in touch with friends and family by phone, Skype, or Zoom. Have plenty of soap, great music, and meditations on hand.

The Coronavirus increases our need for conscientious health care, as described in this book. In fact, the advice I'd give in meeting this pandemic serves as a summary of chapters. You might as well give up on the notion that the federal government will "get it right." Its handling of the pandemic has been militantly ignorant and lacking in common sense. You need to take the initiative in practicing self-care, which includes "social distancing" and other policies/practices aimed at breaking the viral vector transmission: A conscientious person cares for the health of others, as well as the self.

Above all, *your greatest defense is positive thinking.* Time and again we've noted the findings of Dr. Eysenck: that 75% of people who die of cancer have lifelong depression, 15% have lifelong anger, and 9% have both. These stats are mirrored by heart disease: 75% of those who die of heart disease have lifelong anger, 15% have lifelong depression, and 9% have both. For your own health's sake, you cannot afford the luxury of anger, guilt, anxiety, or depression! In the current pandemic, it's critical that you confront your fears or anxiety concerning illness and death. Glance back at the "Stress Management Pocket Card" (illustrated in Chapter 2) and put its advice into practice. Do what you can positively and detach from those things you cannot change.

Here as always, Cayce's general health recommendations are top priority. These include nutrition, exercise, various body therapies, and a positive search for God. Eat fruits and veggies and avoid the junk: That includes the stuff sold for take-out at fast food restaurants, as well as the prepared packed foods sold in supermarkets. Here's a general rule of thumb: If it's packaged in plastic or cardboard, then it's likely junk or toxic. It's time to be reminded that 80% of your diet needs to be alkaline. Well over 90% of our clients come to us with a salivary pH of less than 7. If your salivary pH is consistently acidic, take a heaping teaspoon daily of potassium gluconate powder.

Don't neglect exercise: "Sheltering at home" does not prevent a daily jog, bike ride, or brisk walk outside. If you need to lose weight—and 70% of Americans are overweight, while 35% are downright obese—why not take this time to begin a healthy diet regimen? Same with smoking: 22% of Americans still use tobacco. Now's as good a time as any to stop—it will save you money (and trips to the convenience store). If you're home-bound, now's a perfect time to improve your sleep habits. (If anything, the pandemic may well break us of our workaholism.) Commit to eight luxurious hours of sleep each evening. Give yourself permission to enjoy sleep and look forward to it.

I've already mentioned the search for God and the need for meditation and great music. These contribute to a positive life-attitude; just as important, they contribute to a positive spiritual purpose. Remember the highest purpose of being here on this planet: to help others! Add prayer to mediation. Don't just listen to music, sing it—dance it. Happiness—along with your connection to soul, spirit, and God—is an inside job!

I started this book with a diatribe against water pollution-by-fluoride, so let me end where I began: Through sheer government stupidity, 95% of our drinking water has been poisoned. Fluoride weakens the immune system, calcifies our pineal gland, lowers IQ, and is rapidly sterilizing us. Sperm counts today average 40 million; Sixty years ago it was 150 million. At 20 million, a man is deemed infertile. If we do not get rid of fluoride, within twenty years there will be no new babies. Incidentally, over 50% of bottled water has fluoride in it. (Plastic containers and metal cans, especially those containing carbonated water, are also toxic.) So, even without the threat of Coronavirus, we are staring in the face of a nationwide multivalent epidemic capable of wiping us out.

The CDC and other agencies tell us that people who have chronic disease of any kind are more likely to die if infected with the Coronavirus. And while those over 65 are more likely to die of the virus than are younger Americans, *healthy* octogenarians are likely to outlive *unhealthy* 40-year-olds. In today's toxic world, we need far more than the original "recommended daily allowance" (RDA) of most vitamins. So, now more than ever, it's time to commit to the Shealy-Sorin "basic essentials." All adults should take adequate supplements, including a high potency multivitamin with 25 to 50 mg of the basic B's. Take 50,000 units of vitamin D3 once a week if you weigh 140 pounds or more (and take on the first, tenth, and twentieth of the month if you weigh below 140 pounds).

In this stressful moment, here are some customized commonsense recommendations:[13]

At the "feeling" that a virus is invading your body, take 150,000 units of vitamin D3 three days in a row, and take 15 mg daily of K2.

Take at least 2000 mg of vitamin C daily, preferably with 1000 mg of MSM: These are combined synergistically in Dr. Shealy's Youth Formula. At that feeling of a virus knocking at the door, *double this dosage.* If symptoms worsen, have on hand some liposomal vitamin C and take 5000 to 8000 mg daily. Increase vitamin B6 to 200 mg daily.

A holistic practitioner can administer 25 to 50 grams of vitamin c intravenously in a Myer's cocktail (see Chapter 3). Recently, a New York hospital announced they were treating COVID-19 patients with 1500 mg of vitamin C up to three times daily. They should consider increasing that dose: I've used up to 100 grams of vitamin C in scores of patients.

Take at least 500 mg of beta glucans daily.

Take at least 10 mg of Astaxanthin daily. With the feeling of a virus coming on, increase to 30 mg.

Take 100 mg daily of tocotrienols (vitamin E) daily.

---

13 Note that the following recommendations offer generalized immune support useful in lessening the severity of viral infection. These do not prevent infection from Coronavirus, nor do they "cure" it.

Ozone is another great inhibitor of all infections, including viral. It can be physician-administered by insufflation (blown into the sinuses or ear cavities); it can also be administered intravenously as a blood infusion. I'm pleased to note that ozone treatments have become a specialty of the Shealy-Sorin Wellness Institute.

Detox your body regularly! My favorite detox (described in Chapter 3) is castor oil packs on the abdomen five days a week and at least once a week thereafter. At the feeling of virus invasion, use a castor oil suit. (After bathing, rub castor oil over your entire body from the bottom of your neck to your wrists and ankles. Then wear an old sweat suit to bed.) If a sauna is available, you can instead rub on the castor oil and spend 20 minutes in sauna.

Keep a hair dryer at hand. At the feeling of virus invasion, spray your face with water and cup your hand over half of the intake valve; then, with each breath, inhale the hot air. Do this for five minutes three times daily.

The Sapphire-Enhanced AdrenoScalar is a multipurpose device that reduces free radicals, which are increased in any inflammatory condition. Inflammation is increased by infections like COVID-19. An hour or two daily of AdrenoScalar treatment decreases free radicals by 80%.

Another general health-enhancer is the Shealy-Sorin Gamma PEMF, which improves circulation and reduces inflammation.

The Shealy Bliss oils have their role to play, too. Fire

Bliss raises DHEA, the anti-stress hormone, and is useful in overcoming depression. Earth Bliss raises calcitonin, the essential hormone for bone calcification and decreasing pain. Crystal Bliss reduces free radicals by 80%. And Air Bliss raises oxytocin, the essential hormone in bonding and nurturing.

If you do not already have a daily meditative tool, Autogenic Training (described in Chapters 2-3) is useful in overcoming depression, anxiety, and pain. Biogenics AT trains the brain to detach from those fears you cannot change. Ideally, you should practice AT eighteen minutes twice a day for three months. (And it is useful in 80% of all illnesses!) An mp3 is available free on the Shealy-Sorin Wellness Institute website: www.ShealyWellness.com.

Finally, hospitals and many clinics keep an Impedance Threshold Device (ITD) on hand for CPR. This, along with a Radiac, could be of great value in COVID-19 emergencies.

One of the biggest problems highlighted by the Coronavirus pandemic is the woefully small number of holistic physicians who can administer the sorts of treatment described above. Of course, those who ascribe to Edgar Cayce's Association for Research and Enlightenment—Cayce's A.R.E.—are the best by far!

In sum: Though the current crisis brings hardships for all, it is also the best opportunity offered so far in this century to gain in soul-growth. Do not panic. Thinking sets in motion spiritual forces capable of balancing body, mind, and soul. Think love. Think health. Think hope. Think peace. Think HEAL.

POSTLUDE

Healthy Poetry for the Conscientious

Georgianne S. Ginder, CSE
(Self-Certified Common Sense Expert!)

The Science of the Soul

The science of the soul:
Eternal wisdom that keeps us whole.
We study emotions, body, mind,
And yet ignore the soul.
Have we been rendered blind?

Peace it seems
Is hard to find.
The holistic remedy?
Sustainable spirituality.

Seek the light
The love
The truth—
—In kind:
Know blessings of the ties that bind.

"Blest be the tie that binds.
A fellowship of kindred minds
Is like to that above."

—Georgianne Ginder
(written during a church service, June 2, 2019)

I Have Now to Live

I have *now* to live—
Live in "this space."
I claim no label:
No diagnosis frames me or claims me—
Nor must I own it.

Yet I acknowledge that *matter* "matters" ...
Thoughts move in and (*eventually!*) out
(Thoughts of promise, joy, or doubt).

Voices clamor to be heard.
Beneath each thought, each glimpse, each word
Rests the Divine:
The light, the spark, the sight, the love—
Waiting patiently to be stirred.

—Georgianne Ginder (February 28, 2015)

The Appointed Hour

Each of us at that appointed hour
Will "figuratively" die.

How we proceed
Depends on our projected wants,
Our program
And our learned needs.

Who we are?
How we live?
Seek the Truth or
Accept the lie:

What we strive to get—
And give—
Contributes to the way we die.

Each of us
Does have a choice—
Of ways we use our wisdom,
Our influence, and our voice—

Until that hour when we "'switch" our power—
A harvest grown from root to flower.

—Georgianne Ginder (November 19, 2010)

Chem Tails

(Tales from the Vault of Hush-Hush Assault.
Asthma anyone?)

Back then ...
"Look up to the sky,"
The Old -Timer said,
"And tell me what you see."
"A sky of blue,
A cloud or two,
What it looks like to me."

And now ...
"Scan the sky and tell me why
Those criss-crossed trails are drifting by.
For soon the blue will turn to grey,
Another milky cloud-filled day:
More headaches and wheezing on the way."

Invisible trails, we are patronizingly told,
Cannot!—do not!—exist!
Yet why do skies that tells no lies
Persist, persist, persist?

We breathe that toxic, nano mist
And wonder why most still resist.

The brain is drained of common sense:
Grey matter
Tells the tale:

Look to the sky and ponder why
Not to question is to fail.

The Old -Timer said,
Sadly shaking his head,
"How did it get this way?
They fail to see,
They fail to be—
They cease to find their way."
        —Georgianne Ginder (August 11, 2019)

We Destroy What We Fear

Splendidly it glistened in the sun!
Hours before there had been no hint
Of this symmetry, this growing web
Poised purposely over my back door.

And too the work seemed effortless—
And apparently had just begun.

The spider looked as if to say,
"Good morning, now,
And by the way I have just as much right
To this doorframe as you."
I thought a moment. Was this true?

And so she did.
And what, if anything, would I do?

Observing the birdfeeder, seed in hand,
Greeting the squirrels, a dove, and sparrow,
I looked closely at this new addition
And how it chilled me to the marrow.

Wasn't that an hourglass
Tattooed, it seemed, upon her torso?

Perhaps there is a danger here?
Is this the creature I've been taught to fear?
With broom in hand
I banished the nest to the netherworld,
Crushing the arachnid beneath my shoe.

I said I was sorry as I quashed her life
Beneath me.

I had lost control somehow and yet
I did not know what else to do.
As life evaporated beneath my foot
This awareness again within me grew:

You are safe until I've learned to fear you.
You stay secure until I do.
But once afraid, destruction happens
And precious life can ebb away—
Beneath the sole of any shoe.

—Georgianne Ginder (September 15, 2003)

Poisoned Heels/Poison Heals:
The Words of Wo-De Ke-Ca

In sixth grade (and beyond) at West Elementary School, my Campfire Girls' name was Wo-De Ke-Ca, meaning "Skillful Artist." She was of the clan of Ao-Wa-Kiya, "those who band together for a purpose." Wo-De Ke-Ca speaks to me periodically, as in the following poem:

We poison our earth with impunity, digging our heels in and
carrying out—and carrying on
As if the earth exists as our enemy instead of our home, our
healer.
We fracture our water, our living water, and wonder why we
are such a sickened and cancerous breed.
We poison, alter, and modify our seeds so they longer sustain
us:
We pretend that such toxins and chemical mutations are bene-
ficial to us,
Will make us wiser, healthier, save us money, make life easier,
provide us leisure.
But we are not enjoying life ... for we are foolish and seldom
truly free:
We are exploited as we are exploiting and fail to want to see.
All the while we grow weaker, impoverished, banal, and wor-
ship-full-of greed.
Progress is it called. *Some* call it so. *But I?* I am here now,
Here to awaken you, to remind you, too,
For when we are true to ourselves, *we know.*

We tell ourselves that poison heals,
That chemical cocktails—never before known to humankind, to
animals and plants,
to minerals, water and soil, to any and to all—are good,
That merging man and mouse in the name of research
Will spur that "cure,"
That a "clone" of a cure is wise, and sound and safe and pure.

That chemo "therapies" and the radiation drugs that render us
helpless,
Immune-compromised, toxified in body and soul,
Will buy us "time," will free us from ourselves so we can *beat
death* and live forever!

But I know better.
And so does our Mother Earth, our living lesson, our judicious
and prudent teacher,
Who with our Father God has given us birth. Our Supreme
Highest Power
And other powers—those who are crying out to us, beseeching
us to awaken and to see:
The eagle and dove, the wolf and the sparrow, the butterfly and
bee, the flower and the tree—
Are reminding us of what we are soon to lose.
The rolling waters and whistling winds are warning us.
Yet we are unwilling to slow down and to listen.
We are busy.

We want our progress and we want our sweetbreads and we
long for more and more
To consume, even as we are consumed, eaten alive.

And still we pretend that we are wise,
That nature and nurture must graciously bow to our new and
ever newer science,
While our compliance and reliance go unquestioned and rewarded!

Though deep deep down within our soul-selves we detect (oh
yes, many do)
That we are losing our way and unable virtually unwilling to
find our higher voice;
We suspect that we have abandoned the Wisdom God of all
Times and Places.
We have chosen to ride the road of relentless pursuit of egotis-
tic power.
To poison ourselves appears to make no sense,
And yet we applaud those who are willing to do so,
Who sell their sort of snaking oil, promoting such practices,
pronouncing them "safe and good,"
Who take our monies and experiment upon our lives and live-
lihood,
Our health and wellness, and ask us to continue to trust—
Not to question but to buy in.
And some of us do buy in.

But I?
I have returned to ask you:
Is this wise, or good, or safe, or true?
I ask you
And I await your reply.

I, Princess Wo-De Ke-Ca, return to speak with one and all who
will listen!
Poison does not heal.
Poison clouds, distracts, destroys and deludes.
Wisdom prevails, summons and patiently intrudes.
Time will bear truth for those who are wise enough to wonder,
to wander and to see.
For the rest, who remain asleep—
Poison heals.

Poisoned Heels: The name of those who accept blindness over
the light,
Who live in unquestioning dimness and declare such darkness
safe and good.
Yet there are always those who claim *the sight*.
—Georgianne Ginder (Easter eve, March 26, 2016)

No Fly Zone

End of June
It almost is
And nary a fly I've seen.
A bee?
Make that two—
One butterfly?
What has this come to mean?

Overkill by pesticides,
Such "electro-frequent" fog?

The poisons that pummel and promulgate
Such hazy growing smog.

Am I next?
Have we all been hexed?
Email, snail mail, tweet and text
Mr. Fly,
Fly on by—
I sense your "buzzing" battle cry.

—Georgianne Ginder

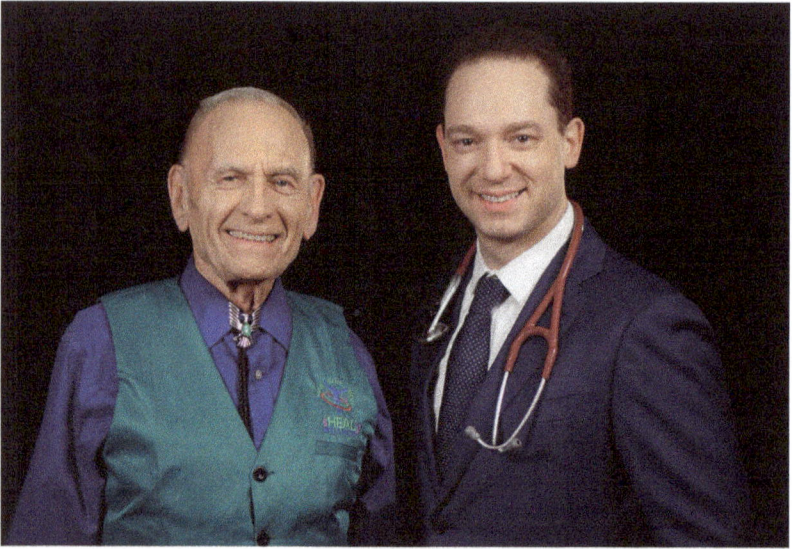

C. Norman Shealy, M.D., Ph.D. and Sergey Sorin, M.D., DABFM

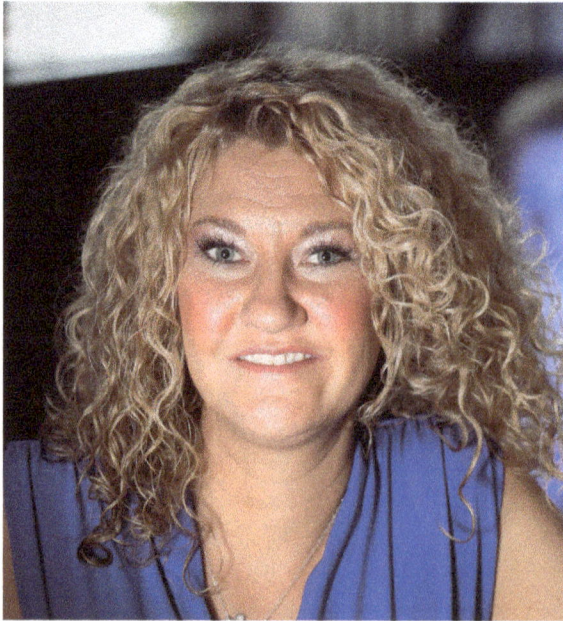

Amber R. Massey-Abernathy, Ph.D.

About the Authors

C. Norman Shealy, M.D., Ph.D. is Founder and President of International Institute of Holistic Medicine, President of Shealy Wellness, LLC and Holos Energy Medicine Education. He is editor of *Journal of Comprehensive Integrative Medicine*. He was founding President of the American Holistic Medical Association in 1978. He was founding President of Holos University Graduate Seminary and is now Professor Emeritus of Energy Medicine. He holds fifteen patents in energy medicine and has published thirty-five books and over 300 articles. For the past twenty-nine years, he has hosted the Shealy Wellness radio show on KWTO in Springfield, Mo.

Sergey Sorin, M.D., DABFM is a Board-certified physician with extensive clinical experience in conventional healthcare, as well as a long history of healthcare leadership. After a life-altering diagnosis and successful holistic treatment of colon cancer in 2007 (in full remission and thriving, despite a poor prognosis from mainstream oncology), his focus has been on the broad field of holistic medicine personally and professionally. His publications include books, articles, and original research projects in peer-reviewed scientific journals. He is a co-host of the Shealy-Sorin Wellness radio show and has been a keynote speaker at numerous national and international conferences. Dr. Sorin is currently CEO and Medical Director of the Shealy-Sorin Wellness Institute, continuing and expanding on the work of C. Norman Shealy, M.D. Ph.D.—one of the true pioneers and founding fathers of the Holistic Movement.

Amber R. Massey-Abernathy, Ph.D., is Associate Professor of Psychology at Missouri State University, where she specializes in psychology of childhood, psychology of adolescence, and personality. Her research in various fields, include stress and the application of Five-Factor Theory, have been published in numerous scholarly journals. She holds the Mary-Charlotte Bayles Shealy Chair in Conscientious Psychology.

Georgianne Ginder, M.Sc., is a JSJ certified practitioner working as a health and wellness counselor for the Health Arts and Healthcare Program at Virginia Commonwealth University. She is a longtime member of the American Holistic Medical Association. Her poems and meditations are regularly featured on the Shealy-Sorin Wellness website.

Appendix:
Products and Resources

Shealy-Sorin Wellness Institute:
2840 E. Chestnut Expressway
Springfield, Missouri 65802
Open 8 a.m. to 5 p.m. Monday through Friday.
Tel: (417) 467-2124
Web: www.ShealyWellness.com
www.realholisticdoc.com

Many of the supplements and all of the Institute's proprietary electromagnetic devices are available online or by telephone. The more popular devices include:
Shealy-Sorin Gamma PEMF
Sapphire-Enhanced AdrenoScalar
RelaxMate II Visual Relavation System
TENS 2000 with timer

For pricing, visit the website, https://normshealy.shop/collections/piezoelectric-healing. In many ways, this present book expands on the holistic philosophy informing *90 Days to Self-Health* and *30 Days to Self-Health*. Those books give more detailed explanations of many of the protocols outlined here, so we recommend them as vital companion pieces to the present work.

The most convenient hotel for out of town clients is GreenStay Hotel and Suites, just two blocks from the Wellness Institute:
222 N Ingram Mill Ave.
Springfield, MO 65802
Tel: (417) 863-1440

Seutermann Homeopathy:

For ordering materials for Seutermann Homeopathy, contact the distributor of Heel products in the United States:

BHI/Biological Homeopathic Industries, Inc.
10421 Research Road SE
Albuquerque, NM 87123
Tel: (800) 621-7644
(505) 275-1672
Fax: (800) 217-6934
Web: HeelUSA.com
Email: info@HeelUSA.com

For an alternative source for Seutermann protocol, contact:
Celletech Inc.
518 Tasman St, Madison, WI 53714
Tel: (800) 888-4066

Autoimmune-X:
PRISTINE NUTRACEUTICALS
2805 E. Oakland Park Blvd., #419
Fort Lauderdale, FL 33306
Tel: (888) 671-2873

The agility
Of the ability
Affords tranquility:

Antidote to hostility!

—Georgianne Ginder

www.ingramcontent.com/pod-product-compliance
Lightning Source LLC
Chambersburg PA
CBHW042248040426
42336CB00043B/3328